PUBLIC HEALTH IN THE 21ST CENTURY

PUBLIC HEALTH EMERGENCY MEDICAL COUNTERMEASURES ENTERPRISE STRATEGY AND IMPLEMENTATION PLAN

Public Health in the 21st Century

Additional books in this series can be found on Nova's website under the Series tab.

Additional E-books in this series can be found on Nova's website under the E-book tab.

PUBLIC HEALTH IN THE 21ST CENTURY

PUBLIC HEALTH EMERGENCY MEDICAL COUNTERMEASURES ENTERPRISE STRATEGY AND IMPLEMENTATION PLAN

NIEL A. HARRIS
EDITOR

nova publishers
New York

For permission to use material from this book please contact us:
Telephone 631-231-7269; Fax 631-231-8175
Web Site: http://www.novapublishers.com

Library of Congress Cataloging-in-Publication Data

ISBN: 978-1-62808-861-8

Published by Nova Science Publishers, Inc. † New York

Contents

PREFACE

The United States continues to face a range of serious threats to its national health security from the deliberate use or accidental release of chemical, biological, radiological, and nuclear (CBRN) agents, as well as from naturally occurring and emerging infectious diseases, including pandemic influenza. A failure to anticipate these threats – or the lack of a capacity to effectively respond to them – could leave an untold number of Americans dead or permanently disabled. The United States must therefore have the nimble, flexible capability to produce and effectively utilize medical countermeasures in the face of any attack or threat whether known or unknown – novel or reemerging – natural or intentional. In addition, these capabilities must be communicated to the American public both before and during an emergency. The Secretary of Health and Human Services (HHS) leads all Federal public health and medical response to public health and medical emergencies covered by the National Response Framework. Effectively fulfilling this responsibility and accomplishing these goals necessitates coordination of medical countermeasure-related activities occurring across multiple Federal departments. To provide this coordination, HHS established the Public Health Emergency Medical Countermeasures Enterprise (PHEMCE) in July 2006 to coordinate Federal efforts to enhance civilian preparedness from a medical countermeasure perspective. The PHEMCE is charged with addressing the needs to produce and make medical countermeasures available to limit potential adverse health impacts on the large and diverse U.S. civilian population. The PHEMCE is working to meet the public health emergency needs of the entire civilian population, including groups that require special medical considerations, such as children and the elderly, as well as for first responders, health personnel, and other critical infrastructure personnel, by taking a "whole of community" approach in planning, response, and recovery efforts.

Chapter 1 – The U.S. Government has a responsibility to protect the health and safety of its citizens. The American people continue to face a host of national health security threats from chemical, biological, radiological, and nuclear (CBRN) agents (e.g., weapons that could be used to kill or injure a large number of people) and emerging infectious diseases (EID) (e.g., 1918-19 influenza pandemic outbreak). Under the leadership of the Department of Health and Human Services (HHS) the Public Health Emergency Medical Countermeasures Enterprise (PHEMCE) is the coordinating body for the federal agencies in charge of protecting the civilian population from potential adverse health impacts through the use of medical countermeasures, which are medicines, devices, or other medical interventions that can lessen the harmful effects of these threats. Since the first PHEMCE Strategy and Implementation Plan were released in 2007, critical medical countermeasures have been developed, acquired, and stockpiled for emergency use. Plans have been made across all levels of government to ensure these critical assets can be used effectively in an emergency. Additionally, experiences ranging from real public health emergencies to national-level exercises have presented opportunities for the PHEMCE to assess medical countermeasure preparedness planning and to reallocate resources based on lessons learned.

Chapter 2 – The *2012 Public Health Emergency Medical Countermeasures Enterprise (PHEMCE) Implementation Plan* describes the priorities that HHS, in collaboration with its interagency partners, will implement over the next five years to advance the strategic goals and underlying objectives established in the *2012 PHEMCE Strategy*. Priorities are identified along the near- (Fiscal Year [FY] 12-14), mid- (FY15-17), and long-term (FY18 and beyond) timeframes where appropriate. Together, the *2012 PHEMCE Strategy* and *Implementation Plan* provide the blueprint for the PHEMCE to enhance national health security through the procurement and use of life-saving medical countermeasures (MCMs). As stated in the *Strategy*, the PHEMCE is driven by two core principles: (1) the medical and public health imperative to limit the potential adverse health impacts posed by a variety of threats, and (2) the fiduciary responsibility to maximize the preparedness that can be gained with the significant but finite resources available. The *Implementation Plan* lays out a prioritization framework that is consistent with these core principles, and seeks to best manage the difficult choices facing the PHEMCE, in light of fiscal constraints, scientific limitations, and other factors. Using this prioritization framework the *Implementation Plan* identifies priority activities across the various PHEMCE mission areas, including requirement-setting; basic research; discovery and early development; advanced development; regulatory science management; procurement and stockpiling; response planning; distribution and dispensing; and monitoring, evaluation, and assessment programs. These priorities support the goals and objectives in the *Strategy*, and are summarized in Table 1. The *Implementation Plan* provides both a broad-based description of these priority activities, as well as further detail regarding threat-based and capabilities-based approaches. The Assistant Secretary for Preparedness and Response (ASPR) will establish an internal tracking mechanism to monitor and evaluate the execution of priorities identified in the *2012 PHEMCE Implementation Plan* and report progress regularly to senior leadership and, to the extent feasible in light of national security and proprietary concerns, to external stakeholders. It is anticipated that the *PHEMCE Strategy* and *Implementation Plan* will be reviewed and updated every five years, or more frequently if needed.

In: Public Health Emergency ...
Editor: Niel A. Harris
ISBN: 978-1-62808-861-8

Chapter 1

2012 Public Health Emergency Medical Countermeasures Enterprise (PHEMCE) Strategy*

U.S. Department of Health and Human Services

Executive Summary

The U.S. Government has a responsibility to protect the health and safety of its citizens. The American people continue to face a host of national health security threats from chemical, biological, radiological, and nuclear (CBRN) agents (e.g., weapons that could be used to kill or injure a large number of people) and emerging infectious diseases (EID) (e.g., 1918-19 influenza pandemic outbreak). Under the leadership of the Department of Health and Human Services (HHS) the Public Health Emergency Medical Countermeasures Enterprise (PHEMCE) is the coordinating body for the federal agencies in charge of protecting the civilian population from potential adverse health impacts through the use of medical countermeasures, which are medicines, devices, or other medical interventions that can lessen the harmful effects of these threats.

Since the first PHEMCE Strategy and Implementation Plan were released in 2007, critical medical countermeasures have been developed, acquired, and

* This is an edited, reformatted and augmented version of the U.S. Department of Health and Human Services, dated 2012.

stockpiled for emergency use. Plans have been made across all levels of government to ensure these critical assets can be used effectively in an emergency. Additionally, experiences ranging from real public health emergencies to national-level exercises have presented opportunities for the PHEMCE to assess medical countermeasure preparedness planning and to reallocate resources based on lessons learned.

Overview of PHEMCE Strategic Goals and Objectives

Goal 1: Identify, create, develop, manufacture and procure critical medical countermeasures.

Objective 1.1: Develop a strategic framework to prioritize PHEMCE resources and investments.

Objective 1.2: Utilize consistent approaches for medical consequence and public health response assessments and medical countermeasure requirement setting that include consideration of effective production, storage, deployment and administration strategies.

Objective 1.3: Ensure a robust and sustainable product pipeline for medical countermeasures that emphasizes multi-functional capabilities rather than stand alone outcomes (e.g., platform technologies, host-based innovations, broad-spectrum medical countermeasures) and includes consideration of viable commercial markets and/or routine public health applicability.

Objective 1.4: Promote effective domestic and international partnerships with developers and manufacturers and support core services.

Goal 2: Establish and communicate clear regulatory pathways to facilitate MCM development and use.

Objective 2.1: Identify scientific and regulatory issues that challenge medical countermeasure development or use during public health emergencies and coordinate activities among PHEMCE partners to address those challenges.

Objective 2.2: Assist medical countermeasure developers in working interactively with FDA during product development and regulatory review.

Goal 3: Develop logistics and operational plans for optimized use of medical countermeasures at all levels of response.

Objective 3.1: Promote innovative approaches to inventory management to enable a sustainable preparedness infrastructure.

Objective 3.2: Develop and communicate medical countermeasure utilization policy, guidance and response strategies, including FDA regulatory frameworks, that are responsive to end-user needs, that are integrated with State, local, tribal and territorial (SLTT) and private sector response plans, and when possible international partners, and that ensure timely, safe, and effective medical countermeasure distribution and utilization.

Objective 3.3: Develop and provide medical countermeasure communications, training, and education information to inform all stakeholders.

Objective 3.4: Develop and implement strategies to assess, evaluate, and monitor medical countermeasure safety, performance, and patient compliance during and after a public health emergency response.

Goal 4: Address medical countermeasure gaps for all sectors of the American civilian population.

Objective 4.1: Develop medical consequence and public health response assessments and requirements setting for at-risk individuals.[1]

Objective 4.2: Support medical countermeasure advanced development and procurement for at-risk individuals.

Objective 4.3: Develop and implement strategies, policies, and guidance to support the appropriate use of medical countermeasures in all civilian populations during an emergency.

Above all, the PHEMCE mission and outputs must preserve and protect people's lives against a wide range of dangerous threats and do so as good stewards of the taxpayer's dollars. These are two core principles of the

PHEMCE Strategy. Standing on past progress and seeking to make the best use of available resources, the *2012 PHEMCE Strategy* establishes these strategic goals for the PHEMCE over the next five years:

- Identify, create, develop, manufacture, and procure critical medical countermeasures.
- Establish and communicate clear regulatory pathways to facilitate medical countermeasure development and use.
- Develop logistics and operational plans for optimized use of medical countermeasures at all levels of response.
- Address medical countermeasure gaps for all sectors of the American civilian population.

PHEMCE Leadership has identified a set of criteria against which all investments must be prioritized. These include (1) addressing the most significant threats, (2) fostering approaches with the potential to provide protection against multiple important threats, and (3) maintaining the capability to effectively use the assets developed in the envisioned operational setting. The 2012 *PHEMCE Implementation Plan*, to be released in summer 2012, will further describe the prioritization of programs based on these criteria. This Strategy and the Implementation Plan together provide the blueprints the PHEMCE will follow in the near, mid-, and long-terms to make the best use of available resources to enhance national health security.

INTRODUCTION

The United States continues to face a range of serious threats to its national health security from the deliberate use or accidental release of chemical, biological, radiological, and nuclear (CBRN) agents, as well as from naturally occurring and emerging infectious diseases, including pandemic influenza. A failure to anticipate these threats – or the lack of a capacity to effectively respond to them – could leave an untold number of Americans dead or permanently disabled. The United States must therefore have the nimble, flexible capability to produce and effectively utilize medical countermeasures[2,3] in the face of any attack or threat whether known or unknown– novel or reemerging – natural or intentional. In addition, these capabilities must be communicated to the American public both before and during an emergency.

The Secretary of Health and Human Services (HHS) leads all Federal public health and medical response to public health and medical emergencies covered by the National Response Framework.[4] A number of National Strategies and Presidential Directives establish HHS as the lead Federal department responsible for the protection of the health of the civilian population against both intentional and accidental or naturally occurring threats.[5] Additionally, the HHS Strategic Plan 2010-2015 calls for reducing the occurrence of infectious diseases, protecting Americans' health and safety during emergencies, and fostering resilience in response to emergencies; these goals are also reflected in particular strategic initiatives set by the Secretary.[6] Effectively fulfilling this responsibility and accomplishing these goals necessitates coordination of medical countermeasure-related activities occurring across multiple Federal departments. To provide this coordination, HHS established the Public Health Emergency Medical Countermeasures Enterprise (PHEMCE)[7] in July 2006 to coordinate Federal efforts to enhance civilian preparedness[8] from a medical countermeasure perspective. The PHEMCE is charged with addressing the needs to produce and make medical countermeasures available to limit potential adverse health impacts on the large and diverse U.S. civilian population. The PHEMCE is working to meet the public health emergency needs of the entire civilian population, including groups that require special medical considerations, such as children and the elderly, as well as for first responders, health personnel, and other critical infrastructure personnel, by taking a "whole of community" approach in planning, response, and recovery efforts.

This is a complex mission space and many Federal agencies have responsibilities that are critical to its success. The PHEMCE is led by the Assistant Secretary for Preparedness and Response (ASPR).[9] Core HHS members are the Director for the Centers for Disease Control and Prevention (CDC), the Director of the National Institute of Allergy and Infectious Diseases (NIAID) within the National Institutes of Health (NIH), and the Commissioner of the Food and Drug Administration (FDA). Key PHEMCE interagency partners include senior leadership from the Department of Veterans Affairs (VA), the Department of Defense (DoD), the Department of Homeland Security (DHS), and the U.S. Department of Agriculture (USDA). Additionally the PHEMCE works with appropriate HHS and U.S. Government partners to consider international aspects of its mission when appropriate. The PHEMCE also works closely with a variety of non- Federal partners including State, local, tribal and territorial governments, public health systems, academia, private industry, and ultimately the American people.

The PHEMCE mission is to advance national preparedness for natural, accidental, and intentional threats by coordinating medical countermeasure-related efforts within HHS and in cooperation with PHEMCE interagency partners. The PHEMCE provides a governance structure to achieve this coordination (described in Appendix 3).

The PHEMCE mission components include:

- *Requirements Setting*: The PHEMCE is responsible for establishing requirements for civilian medical countermeasures based on many factors, including threat and risk assessments. DHS is the lead in conducting the threat and risk assessments that are leveraged in PHEMCE requirements setting. ASPR leads the requirements-setting process with engagement from all PHEMCE partners and expert inputs, including medical consequence and public health response assessments.
- *Early Stage Research*: NIH conducts and supports basic research to better understand threats of civilian public health concern. This research provides the foundation for developing medical products and strategies to diagnose, treat, and prevent a wide range of threats. DoD and USDA also conduct early stage research that is pertinent to the PHEMCE mission.
- *Advanced Development/Manufacturing*: ASPR/BARDA is the lead PHEMCE partner supporting advanced development and scale up of manufacturing capacity for medical countermeasures, including promoting partnerships with developers and manufacturers. DoD and USDA also conduct advanced development that is coordinated and leveraged through the PHEMCE.
- *Regulatory Science Management*: The PHEMCE conducts regulatory science[10] to facilitate medical countermeasure development, regulatory assessment, and use. The FDA is the lead agency charged with ensuring medical countermeasures are safe and effective. Activities conducted in support of this mission component intersect with many other mission components in product development and utilization.
- *Procurement/Inventory Management/Stockpiling*: The PHEMCE oversees the procurement of medical countermeasures and their associated inventory management, including stockpiling. Both the CDC and ASPR/BARDA have lead roles in procuring medical countermeasures for stockpiling. The CDC leads the procurement and

maintenance of commercially available medical countermeasures for stockpiling in the Strategic National Stockpile (SNS). BARDA procures certain medical countermeasures for the SNS using the Special Reserve Fund (SRF) authorized under the Project BioShield Act of 2004. DoD and the Department of Veterans' Affairs may also serve as needed in planning or executing stockpiling options.

- *Response Planning, Policy, Guidance and Communication*: The CDC and ASPR coordinate the development of Federal response plans, policy, guidance, and communication, and develop clinical utilization and allocation strategies as appropriate for medical countermeasures and assets. DoD, DHS, and VA are key PHEMCE partners in this mission component.
- *Deployment/Distribution/Dispensing/Administration*: The CDC and ASPR coordinate interactions with State, local, tribal, territorial (SLTT), and private entities to provide timely and effective deployment, distribution, dispensing, and administration of medical countermeasures in an emergency. The VA is a key PHEMCE partner in this mission component.
- *Monitoring/Evaluation/Assessment*: The CDC and FDA lead efforts to monitor safety and performance of deployed medical countermeasures during and after an emergency response. Other PHEMCE partners such as NIH can provide additional capability for clinical trials management or other support roles in evaluation of safety and performance.

A periodic assessment of strategy and capabilities in light of changing scientific and fiscal circumstances is appropriate. Difficult choices must be made to manage risk in ways that favor success in meeting a public health emergency. To this end, HHS updates PHEMCE Strategy and Implementation Plans every five years or more often if needed. The 2007 *PHEMCE Strategy and Implementation Plan for Chemical, Biological, Radiological, and Nuclear (CBRN) Threats,* while acknowledging the complete PHEMCE mission space, predominantly focused on advanced development and acquisition priorities for medical countermeasures using funds available in the Special Reserve Fund authorized under the Project BioShield Act of 2004.[11] The *2012 PHEMCE Strategy* and its related *Implementation Plan* (to be released in summer 2012) are broader in scope, establishing priorities throughout the PHEMCE mission space. Moreover, they address medical countermeasure planning and policies for pandemic influenza and other emerging infectious diseases (in addition to the intentional CBRN threats previously covered in the 2007 effort). The *2012 PHEMCE Strategy* is intended to guide PHEMCE activities for the next five years.

Fulfilling the PHEMCE mission will also require balanced investments in consideration of the long-term sustainability of the Enterprise. Toward this end, the HHS Secretary is also implementing a five year budget planning process across the HHS components of the PHEMCE in order to achieve closer coordination and prioritization of investments in public health emergency preparedness that will be tied to the framework provided by this Strategy. In general this Strategy provides a framework for clarifying priorities, improving decision analysis, and enhancing planning, budgeting, and evaluation activities throughout the PHEMCE.

ACCOMPLISHMENTS SINCE 2007

The *2007 PHEMCE Strategy and Implementation Plan for CBRN Threats* described advanced development and acquisition priorities for CBRN medical countermeasures. Consonant with these plans, seven new critical medical countermeasures have been delivered to the Strategic National Stockpile (SNS) or are in the process of delivery. These medical countermeasures address threats including anthrax, smallpox, botulism toxin, and radiological and nuclear agents. They will allow HHS to better respond to public health emergencies caused by intentional threats or natural events, ultimately saving lives and reducing illness. A brief summary of the key CBRN advanced development and acquisition accomplishments since 2007 with respect to these priorities is shown in Appendix 4. In addition to these accomplishments other notable examples of medical countermeasure advancements include:

- National preparedness levels for botulism were greatly enhanced through completion of stockpile delivery of a new botulinum antitoxin. This new antitoxin is currently used for treatment of sporadic, naturally occurring cases of botulism in the U.S.
- The clinical trial infrastructure developed for biodefense applications was used to support essential clinical studies required for licensure of the 2009 H1N1 vaccines.
- State and local preparedness activities have improved, including laboratory capabilities and response readiness planning for medical countermeasures distribution.[12] For example, CDC has assisted

planning by Cities Readiness Initiative (CRI) participants which has evolved from single hazard, agency-centric plans to all-hazards multi-agency and private partnership plans.
- FDA has issued critical guidance documents that have helped clarify certain pathways to medical countermeasure regulatory approval[13].

In the aggregate, these PHEMCE accomplishments have greatly enhanced our public health emergency preparedness for a wide range of threats and scenarios, and have informed the future directions of the PHEMCE.

CHANGES TO THE MEDICAL COUNTERMEASURE LANDSCAPE

Since the initial *PHEMCE Strategy* and *Implementation Plan* documents were published in 2007, there have been many changes to the medical countermeasure landscape, including the advancements summarized above. Experiences ranging from real public health emergencies to national-level exercises have presented opportunities for the PHEMCE to assess medical countermeasure preparedness planning and to reallocate resources based on lessons learned. For example:

- A recent national-level tabletop exercise of an anthrax attack on a major American city highlighted the need for increased planning to address pediatric prophylaxis needs following an anthrax incident and to better develop and articulate anthrax vaccine allocation guidelines.
- The March 2011 Fukushima–Dai'ichi nuclear power plant incident highlighted that ready access to available medical countermeasures is a major component of public health and safety responses to address such incidents, as well as the importance of international considerations for medical countermeasure utilization policies. This incident additionally emphasized the importance of appropriate and accurate risk messaging to the surrounding populations following catastrophic events as well as the connectivity of the global community in the face of disaster.
- The 2009 H1N1 influenza pandemic demonstrated that, while current medical countermeasure capabilities enabled a robust national response, there remain continuing needs to accelerate and improve

disease detection capabilities, medical countermeasure development production, and distribution capabilities, and the process by which limited medical countermeasures are allocated. Additionally, the pandemic response exposed world-wide gaps in detection and response capabilities and tested the ability of the World Health Organization (WHO) in collaboration with developed countries, including the U.S., to respond to international requests for antivirals and vaccine. Together these highlighted the importance of U.S. Government support for building global capacity for medical countermeasure development and use, including U.S. deployment of medical countermeasures internationally during emergencies, where appropriate.

New national strategic plans have greatly influenced the PHEMCE and our understanding of what it means to be prepared with regard to medical countermeasures. The 2009 release of a quadrennial National Health Security Strategy and the later released Implementation Plan by HHS addresses many aspects of public health emergency preparedness, including the important role of medical countermeasures, and the PHEMCE is aligning its efforts moving forward with the goals articulated here. Also, Presidential Policy Directive 8 on national preparedness, released in 2011, provided further direction aimed at strengthening the security and resilience of the United States by preparing for threats that pose the greatest risk to the security of the Nation, including acts of terrorism, pandemics, and catastrophic natural disasters.[14]

Our medical countermeasures development capability was called out for review by the HHS Secretary in response to the 2009 H1N1 influenza pandemic and other response and planning efforts. Her charge to identify needed improvements resulted in a series of new infrastructure initiatives and enhancements to expand our nation's capacity to respond quickly and effectively to CBRN and emerging infectious disease threats and to support regulatory innovation, domestic manufacturing capacity, and PHEMCE-wide management and effectiveness.[15] President Obama in his 2010 State of the Union message also called for "launching a new initiative that will give [the United States] the capacity to respond faster and more effectively to bioterrorism or an infectious disease—a plan that will counter threats at home, and strengthen public health abroad." These improvements are being pursued actively and are integrated into the current PHEMCE Strategy.

Additionally, HHS has made great strides in implementing the Public Readiness and Emergency Preparedness (PREP) Act[16] authorities and continues to leverage and exercise its use of these authorities. The PREP Act authorizes the Secretary to provide liability immunity to medical countermeasure developers, manufacturers, distributors, program planners, and other qualified persons who prescribe, administer, or dispense covered countermeasures during or in anticipation of a public health emergency. Moreover, the PREP Act authorizes compensation for certain injuries resulting from the use of these countermeasures. HHS has repeatedly heard from stakeholders that liability protection is a necessary incentive for them to undertake activities to develop, manufacture, distribute, and dispense critical countermeasures. The protections provided under the PREP Act ensure that certain barriers (including the unavailability or prohibitive cost of liability insurance) do not limit the availability of critical countermeasures in a public health emergency.

Finally, significant investments have been made by HHS and its interagency partners in the medical countermeasure mission. Given currently available resources from the Federal to the state, local, tribal and territorial levels (SLTT) and existing public health infrastructure, the PHEMCE must work to ensure long-term sustainability of the mission, while maintaining and building a national capability to respond to national security threats. This includes assessing risks and establishing and communicating clear priorities, collaborating closely with SLTT partners, seeking multi-use solutions wherever possible, and working to develop innovative development, manufacturing, stockpiling, and fielding alternatives.

DEVELOPMENT OF THE 2012 PHEMCE STRATEGY

ASPR led the development of the 2012 PHEMCE Strategy through an interagency steering committee comprised of representatives from across the PHEMCE agencies. The steering committee reviewed existing strategies, implementation plans, and other documents with direct relevance to setting PHEMCE goals and objectives. The PHEMCE-wide strategic goals and objectives identified in this Strategy are consistent with these previously identified, agency-level strategies and priorities. Following review and input from across the PHEMCE, the Strategy was approved by HHS and publically released.

Strategic Prioritization Framework

Two core principles guide the activities of the PHEMCE and are reflected in the strategic goals and objectives presented in this document:

- *Limit Adverse Health Impacts* – The ultimate benefit of investing in medical countermeasure preparedness activities is to limit the adverse health effects impacts (deaths, illness, etc.) caused by CBRN and naturally occurring threats to national health security. Programmatic prioritization will take into consideration the potential for each product or program to ultimately prevent fatalities and/or reduce morbidity, including the capability to address the needs of at-risk populations.
- *Stewardship of Resources that create an enduring capability* – To achieve our vision of a responsive and flexible capability to provide medical countermeasures for all hazards, it is important to create a sustainable assemblage of products and supporting infrastructure to reliably get the products to the point of need, especially as financial resources become more constrained. Enduring capability here captures both fiscal and operational meanings. Good stewardship of taxpayer resources demands that the PHEMCE identify and foster products or technologies that serve more than one purpose or that are less reliant on government-only sources of support where possible. The potential for commercial viability (e.g., use in routine public health and/or medical applications), advancement of platform technologies, and innovative, effective, and efficient approaches to inventory management and operational improvements that enhance life-cycle management of medical countermeasures are examples of avenues that help to strengthen the sustainability of the PHEMCE, and these will be considered when establishing program priorities.

Because resources are finite, and there are still a number of important needs, the PHEMCE must have a compelling and transparent set of criteria for assessing all investment decisions. PHEMCE Leadership has identified a strategic framework comprising three essential criteria against which all investments are to be prioritized. These include (1) the need to focus predominantly on addressing the most significant threats; (2) give greater priority to approaches, products, or technologies that are multi-functional; and

(3) foster products that improve our ability to ease operational burdens in distribution and dispensing products to the end-user. PHEMCE leadership will thus apply these criteria to guide decisions on programmatic prioritization across the Enterprise:

1. The PHEMCE must still address the most significant threats (see list of high-priority threats in Box 1 below); however, significant progress has been made against anthrax, smallpox, and botulinum toxin, and while improvements to existing countermeasures are needed, a shifting of focus over time to the remaining threats is warranted.
2. The PHEMCE is in a transition point, moving from products that address single threats to a more agile and sustainable system that has the potential for expanded coverage of threats and that may provide capability against unknown pathogens. It will therefore be important to prioritize efforts when and where possible that provide this capability (e.g., broad-spectrum, multi-functional, platform approaches).
3. A key PHEMCE focus must be to address end-user needs by clearly developing and communicating the concept of operations under which medical countermeasures will be used.

The *PHEMCE Implementation Plan* will further detail how these principles and criteria are further developed to assess investments for decisions about current and future products.

PHEMCE Strategic Goals and Objectives

The following strategic goals and objectives will guide the policies and decisions of PHEMCE agencies to promote medical countermeasure capabilities that enhance preparedness for CBRN and emerging infectious disease threats to national health security, including pandemic influenza.

GOAL 1. Identify, create, develop, manufacture and procure critical medical countermeasures.

Objective 1.1. Develop a strategic framework to prioritize PHEMCE resources and investments.

BOX 1: HIGH-PRIORITY THREATS

The PHEMCE will continue to address medical countermeasure needs to protect against the following high priority threats which have been determined by the Secretary of Homeland Security to pose a material threat sufficient to affect national security and/or which have the potential to seriously threaten national health security:

- *Bacillus anthracis* (anthrax)*
- Clostridium botulinum toxin (botulism)*
- Cyanide
- Emerging infectious diseases (including pandemic influenza)
- Gram negative organisms
  - *Francisella tularensis* (tularemia)
  - *Yersinia pestis* (plague)
  - *Burkolderia mallei* (glanders) and B. *pseudomallei* (meliodosis)
  - *Rickettsia prowazekii* (typhus)
- Multi-drug resistant *Bacillus anthracis* (MDR anthrax)
- Nerve agents
- Radiological agents (e.g., radiological dispersal devices)
- Nuclear agents
- Variola virus (smallpox)*
- Viral Hemorrhagic Fevers
  - Marburg
  - Ebola

* As significant progress accrues for these threats there will be greater attention paid to the next most important agents over time.

Effective use of medical countermeasures in a public health response is in part dependent on strategic decisions in research and development, manufacturing, and acquisition of medical countermeasures. Additionally, given the range of potential threats and the limited resources available to address them, prioritization of HHS and PHEMCE-wide resources across the medical countermeasure development, acquisition, and utilization continuum is necessary. The PHEMCE will employ a coordinated, strategic framework through which to focus investments across the PHEMCE mission space and will apply this framework to inform resource allocations for research, development, manufacturing, and procurement.

Objective 1.2. Utilize consistent approaches for medical consequence and public health response assessments and medical countermeasure requirement setting that include consideration of effective production, storage, deployment and administration strategies.

Simply stated, PHEMCE medical countermeasure requirements must address the questions of "Who needs what, when, and how?" They serve to improve the outcome of public health emergencies by focusing federal investments toward an aligned research, advanced development, acquisition, deployment, and use agenda by HHS agencies. Moreover, requirements inform private industry and academia about the civilian medical countermeasure needs and facilitate effective coordination of programs with PHEMCE interagency partners.

PHEMCE medical countermeasure requirements will continue to be informed by medical consequence and public health response assessments of the number of people who would likely benefit from being prophylaxed, diagnosed, or treated with a particular medical countermeasure under multiple planning scenarios. These estimates will continue to be vetted by Federal subject matter experts from across the PHEMCE in areas including microbiology, health physics, chemistry, toxicology, medicine, medical care, diagnostics, and by non-federal experts where needed and appropriate.

Medical countermeasure requirements will also continue to be informed by consultations with partners both within and beyond the Federal government to ensure that these requirements are based upon a sound understanding of the Concepts of Operations under which the medical countermeasures will be used. Such medical countermeasure requirements will inform development of countermeasures that can be safely and effectively used following a public health emergency and that will ultimately meet the needs of the American people.

Objective 1.3. Ensure a robust and sustainable product pipeline for medical countermeasures that emphasizes multi-functional capabilities rather than stand alone outcomes (e.g., platform technologies, host-based innovations, broad-spectrum medical countermeasures) and includes consideration of viable commercial markets and/or routine public health applicability.

A robust product pipeline is one in which the number of product candidates in the research and development process is sufficient to assure a high probability of successfully developing a candidate with sufficient safety and efficacy information to support FDA approval[17] for the desired indication(s). The PHEMCE will seek to maintain robust product pipelines where they exist and to build them in areas where critical gaps still remain. The PHEMCE will take a portfolio management approach to ensure that research and development activities are well- coordinated across agencies.

To ensure the enduring capabilities of the Enterprise over time, the PHEMCE will pursue wherever possible medical countermeasures that can address multiple high-priority threats and/or have routine public health applications (and thus commercial viability). The Enterprise is mindful that a "one bug, one drug" or fixed defense[18] approach for medical countermeasure development is still required for some of the highest priority threats, such as anthrax and smallpox. However, a broad-spectrum approach, where scientifically well-supported, may offer more effective and efficient capabilities to address both known and unknown threats. Multi-use products such as broad-spectrum therapeutics and multiplex diagnostic platforms support response in a public health emergency and could also provide routine medical and public health benefits that enhance both the sustainability of the medical countermeasure mission and improve daily national health security.

Objective 1.4. Promote effective domestic and international partnerships with developers and manufacturers and support core services.

Financial and technical partnerships among government, developers, and manufacturers can help foster business sustainability and diversify business risk for private companies and non- profit organizations. Engaging international partners offers opportunities to leverage respective national and international proficiency and expertise to collectively address shortfalls and challenges in the CBRN medical countermeasure development area. Such partnerships are also crucial to create incentives and synergies for facilitating novel, nimble, and innovative solutions to complex problems. Government scientists from across HHS and its interagency partners will continue to work with developers, beginning at the early stages of development, to anticipate and resolve problems that could create bottlenecks in the process.

The PHEMCE will seek to provide core services such as expertise in FDA regulatory affairs, product development, scale-up and manufacturing, and manufacturing capacity. Such services, while critical to the success of the

PHEMCE mission, are often beyond the resources of many individual private entities.

GOAL 2. Establish and communicate clear pathways to facilitate medical countermeasure development and use.

Reducing regulatory uncertainties is critical for fostering medical countermeasure development and availability. Regulatory oversight of medical product development for these high consequence but low frequency events includes both the stewardship that the government exercises to assure products are safe and effective, as well as the operating conditions established to ensure safe and secure access to work involving the threat agents themselves. This presents a complicated landscape for product development that the PHEMCE partners have worked to steadily address. The PHEMCE will continue support for regulatory science to develop new tools, standards, and approaches to accelerate the development and approval of a wide range of medical countermeasures for both emergency response and daily health needs, while maintaining the high standards for safety and efficacy that the American people expect.

Objective 2.1. Identify scientific and regulatory issues that challenge medical countermeasure development or use during public health emergencies and coordinate activities among PHEMCE partners to address those challenges.

The regulatory assessment of medical countermeasures by FDA for approval, clearance, licensure, or authorization[19] is data-driven. However, there are often gaps in scientific knowledge that impede or prevent thorough assessment. These gaps in knowledge arise from multiple sources including intrinsic uncertainties about the biologic behavior of threat agents in potential public health emergencies, as well as from insufficient drug development tools, such as animal models, for creating the necessary data to support regulatory decision-making. Discrepancies in available scientific information and tools result in regulatory uncertainties that many developers perceive as contributing to a higher-than-typical risk environment for engaging in medical countermeasure development.

The FDA, through its Medical Countermeasures Initiative (MCMi), is actively engaged with PHEMCE partners in identifying regulatory and scientific challenges that impede medical countermeasure development and use for high-priority medical countermeasures.[20] The PHEMCE will coordinate and prioritize its activities to resolve these challenges based on near-, mid-, and long-term medical countermeasure priorities and requirements established through the PHEMCE coordinated strategic framework.

Objective 2.2. Assist medical countermeasure developers in working interactively with FDA during product development and regulatory review.

Most of the developers engaged in medical countermeasure development are small biotechnology companies that bring a nimble and innovative approach to the development of new products. However, these companies are often challenged by their limited experience in taking a product through advanced development to FDA licensure, approval, or clearance. For example, these companies often lack experience with animal testing, assay development, product manufacturing, clinical trials, and navigating the regulatory process. For companies without existing infrastructure in these areas, accessing specialized services is difficult and expensive.

PHEMCE partners, in particular the National Institute of Allergy and Infectious Diseases (NIAID) within NIH, BARDA, DoD, and FDA, will continue to provide assistance to medical countermeasure developers in working interactively with FDA throughout the regulatory process to facilitate medical countermeasure development, regulatory assessment, and use. The PHEMCE will ensure these efforts are coordinated, consistent, and accurate.

GOAL 3. Develop logistics and operational plans for optimized use of medical countermeasures at all levels of response.

The Nation must be prepared to appropriately use medical countermeasures in an emergency. This requires robust relationships among Federal planners and the SLTT stakeholders who would ultimately be at the operational edge of a public health emergency response. This includes development of optimal approaches for medical countermeasure inventory management and of plans, policies, procedures, and guidance to ensure timely, safe, and effective medical countermeasure distribution and utilization. This will also require administrative preparedness to ensure that fiscal and administrative authorities and practices that govern the funding, procurement, contracting, hiring, and legal capabilities necessary to mitigate, respond to, and recover from public health threats and emergencies can be accelerated, modified, streamlined, and accountably managed at all levels of government. Achieving these objectives will require communications, training, and education with response stakeholders and ultimately with the American people. In addition, strategies should be developed to evaluate and monitor the use, safety and performance of medical countermeasures during a response – to allow adjustment of operations as needed.

Objective 3.1. Promote innovative approaches to inventory management to enable a sustainable preparedness infrastructure.

An effective national response to a public health emergency requires the capability to provide medical countermeasures to mitigate morbidity and mortality in a clinically relevant time frame. The SNS is the Federal medical countermeasure repository designed to supplement and re- supply State and local public health agencies if locally-held or commercial supplies are depleted during a public health emergency or to provide emergency medical countermeasures not available commercially. Medical countermeasure development must take into account product characteristics that will affect logistical and operational issues. Key product characteristics that affect these options include:

- storage requirements (e.g., room temperature, refrigerated, or frozen),
- transportation requirements,
- packaging and space requirements,
- associated ancillary supplies for administration,
- shelf-life,
- dosage forms for administration (e.g., tablets, suspensions, or injectables), and
- commercial applications (e.g., availability in the supply chain and alternative inventory management systems).

Currently the SNS employs several inventory management mechanisms including stockpile- managed inventory, where resources are held in private sector warehouses on behalf of the SNS, and vendor-managed inventory, in which supplies are rotated by the vendor through normal commercial supply chains. Alternative models of inventory management may also be appropriate in reducing the cost of stockpiling for specific medical countermeasures, notably those that are widely used in the daily U.S. pharmaceutical supply chain.

The PHEMCE will continue to evaluate medical countermeasure candidates for storage under alternative inventory management models and will explore the conditions where alternative models are robust and tested, where these may reduce life-cycle costs and improve the sustainability of the SNS. The PHEMCE will also continue to explore alternative strategies to supplement pre-event medical countermeasure stockpiling, including consideration of "just-in-time" production and/or procurement possibilities, especially for those situations where such mechanisms may provide sufficient medical countermeasure preparedness and significantly reduced costs over time.

Objective 3.2. Develop and communicate medical countermeasure utilization policy, guidance and response strategies, including FDA regulatory frameworks, that are responsive to end-user needs and that are integrated with SLTT and private sector response plans, and when possible international partners, and that ensure timely, safe, and effective medical countermeasure distribution and utilization.

The success of the PHEMCE will be measured by the ability to quickly, safely, and effectively utilize medical countermeasures and to effectively develop, communicate, and provide guidance and education on the role of medical countermeasures in a public health emergency response. SLTT public health and health care systems face reduced funding and greater demands in general and for public health preparedness activities. The PHEMCE will seek to support SLTT authorities by ensuring that Federal medical countermeasure emergency response plans are flexible enough to fit into SLTT and private response partners' activities. The plans will also be standardized sufficiently to facilitate a rapid and effective response across all regions.

The decline in resources for public health preparedness activities and the need for capacity to distribute and utilize medical countermeasures is a challenge to the global community. The 2009 influenza pandemic exposed world-wide gaps in making vaccines and antivirals available for the global population in a timely fashion. The PHEMCE will support development of, to the extent possible and commensurate with U.S. national health security objectives, a collaboration framework with international organizations (like WHO) and partner countries for mutual assistance, harmonized preparedness plans, and guidance for international medical countermeasure distribution and utilization policies.

The PHEMCE will continue to drive product development and use practices by gaining input up- front and on a regular basis from key stakeholders at all levels and from multiple communities of interest both domestically and internationally. The PHEMCE will seek to further develop and strengthen the feedback loop between the end-users and developers of critical medical countermeasures. This will help support consideration by medical countermeasure developers of the most up-to-date information regarding the circumstances under which their products may be used in the field.

PHEMCE members and partners will identify opportunities to improve statutory, regulatory, and policy mechanisms with respect to medical countermeasure distribution, administration, and use.

Objective 3.3. Develop and provide medical countermeasure communications, training, and education information to inform all stakeholders.

The PHEMCE will continue to focus attention on ensuring that accurate evidence and science- based information and training are provided on the use of medical countermeasures during a public health emergency. The best practices in risk communication will be employed in providing medical countermeasure-specific communications that include relevant health information, response plans, and timing, and specific instructions regarding medical countermeasure use. The PHEMCE will enhance transparency and communication on policies regarding priorities for allocation of potentially limited medical countermeasures and overarching response strategies to assist partners and the American people in their preparedness and planning efforts.

Previous risk-communication and engagement activities show that the American people are willing to educate themselves on what to do in case of a public health emergency when the information is provided in a usable and trusted way. As demonstrated in past national emergencies, a prepared and engaged population creates less dependencies and can help PHEMCE partners focus resources on those most in need. The PHEMCE will ensure provision of well-defined and concise guidance, policies, and recommendations that support clear, accurate, and effective communication the American people can trust.

Objective 3.4. Develop and implement strategies to assess, evaluate, and monitor medical countermeasure safety, performance, and patient compliance during and after a public health emergency response.

Optimal use of medical countermeasures in an emergency response situation requires rapid feedback on how well these interventions are working to protect individuals and their families. This information may be used to inform real-time refinement of clinical utilization policies during the response. The availability of this information can also allow public health officials and medical professionals to adjust their medical response strategies as needed. Monitoring systems and processes are critical for the success of the PHEMCE. To be effective, a monitoring system must take into account the demands of patient care in hospital and other emergency settings that may limit the resources available for data gathering and reporting activities; the system should also address the ways that acute care record-keeping could contribute to needed data generation, gathering, and analysis which in turn could help to improve patient care during as well as after the emergency. The PHEMCE will coordinate Federal development and implementation of tools and standards for tracking medical countermeasure performance and adjusting the emergency response in real-time as needed. This includes utilization of the SNS Inventory Tracking and Management System and NIH research centers to evaluate the safety, performance, and uptake of medical countermeasures used during public health emergencies.

GOAL 4. Address medical countermeasure gaps for all sectors of the American civilian population.

At-risk individuals,[21] who make up a significant proportion of the American civilian population at any given time, may have diverse and unique vulnerabilities and medical countermeasure needs. The PHEMCE remains fully committed to working towards the goal of protecting the U.S. population, including at-risk individuals, from intentional threats, pandemic influenza, and other emerging infectious diseases posing a threat to national health security. The following objectives outline how the PHEMCE will work toward better addressing and more fully integrating the needs of at-risk individuals into the medical countermeasure planning and acquisition processes – with the ultimate goal of protecting the whole spectrum of the American population in the event of a public health emergency.

Objective 4.1. Develop medical consequence and public health response assessments and requirements setting for at-risk individuals.

The PHEMCE will increase consideration of and efforts to address the medical countermeasure needs of all individuals from across the various sectors of our population that have specific vulnerabilities or needs. These specific vulnerabilities and medical needs must be included in the medical consequence and public health response assessments that inform medical countermeasure requirements determinations within the PHEMCE. Specific vulnerabilities and medical needs include those of pediatric, geriatric, and obstetric populations, as well as people with chronic medical conditions or compromised immune systems.

Objective 4.2. Support medical countermeasure advanced development and procurement for at-risk individuals.

Investment in emergency medical countermeasure development for these populations has not been feasible for industry without the assistance of the U.S. government due to inherent business risks and ethical and regulatory challenges. The needs of at-risk populations pose challenges to the development and acquisition of medical countermeasures specifically formulated for these groups. The PHEMCE will continue to support evaluation of those medical countermeasures currently held in the SNS for use in these important segments of our population, as well as development of additional dosage forms where needed,[22] including maximizing use of medical countermeasure dosage forms that are suitable for use in multiple populations. PHEMCE organizations will continue to support development-specific indications on medical countermeasures for at-risk populations.

Objective 4.3. Develop and implement strategies, policies, and guidance to support the appropriate use of medical countermeasures in all civilian populations during an emergency.

People in at-risk populations must have coordinated and equitable access to medical countermeasures during public health emergencies. The PHEMCE will seek to ensure that Federal medical countermeasure emergency response plans consider the particular needs of these populations and are based on available medical countermeasure safety and efficacy data in those populations.

Implementation of the Strategy

This *2012 PHEMCE Strategy* reflects the HHS commitment, in collaboration with its interagency partners in the PHEMCE, to provide the Nation with a nimble, flexible capacity to produce medical countermeasures rapidly in the face of any public health attack or threat, known or unknown. For the ultimate benefit of limiting adverse health effects to be realized, the PHEMCE must also be committed to ensuring that medical countermeasures are available and can be effectively and safely utilized by all populations in need. The Strategy provides strategic direction to the Department, signals the Department's intents and priorities to its governmental and private partners, and guides the development of the *2012 PHEMCE Implementation Plan*.

The *2012 PHEMCE Implementation Plan* will be released in summer 2012 and will detail those programs and initiatives throughout the Department that will be prioritized in pursuit of the goals and objectives presented in this document. Both documents together constitute the blueprints the PHEMCE will follow in the near-, mid-, and long-terms to make the best use of available resources to contribute to national health security.

Appendix 1 – Glossary

At-Risk Population	At- risk individuals have needs in one or more of the following functional areas: communication, medical care, maintaining independence, supervision, and transportation. At-risk groups may include children, senior citizens, and pregnant women as well as people who have disabilities, live in institutionalized settings, are from diverse cultures, have limited English proficiency or are non-English speaking, are transportation disadvantaged, have chronic medical disorders, or have pharmacological dependency.
Capabilities-Based Approach or Planning	Preparing, under uncertainty, to provide agile systems across the PHEMCE components suitable for a wide range of known and unknown threats while working within an economic framework that necessitates prioritization in order to provide medical countermeasures in a timely manner and reduce adverse health impact of an emergency.
Consequence Assessment	The process of identifying or evaluating the potential or actual effects of an event, incident, or occurrence.
Core Services	Expertise and capabilities required to overcome the technical, regulatory, manufacturing, commercialization, and business challenges inherent in moving innovative medical countermeasures

	from laboratory to commercial scale production and through the regulatory approval process.
Deployment	To station people and/or pharmaceuticals systematically to an area or during an event.
Dispensing	The process of providing medical countermeasures from points of dispensing (PODs) or other sources directly to individuals or targeted populations in the community in various medical or potentially non-medical settings.
Distribution	The transport and delivery of medical countermeasures from SNS locations to state and regional Receipt, Staging and Storage (RSS) sites, and from RSS locations to points of dispensing (PODs) or other local sites that will handle dispensing to individuals.
Emerging Infectious Diseases (EID)	Emerging infectious diseases include "newly-emerging" infectious diseases (i.e., infectious diseases that heretofore had not been recognized in humans but that could pose a public health risk) and "re-emerging" infectious diseases (i.e., infectious diseases that have been recognized in humans but are increasing in incidence or geographic range), the emergence of which would threaten national health security and require a Federal response to ensure community resiliency.
Material Threat Assessment (MTA)	A DHS-led assessment that includes the number of individuals likely to be exposed to a threat agent in a plausible, high-consequence scenario. Formerly known as a Population Threat Assessment (PTA).
Material Threat Determination (MTD)	Issued by the Secretary of Homeland Security for threat agents deemed to pose a material threat sufficient to affect national security. The MTD is necessary, but not sufficient, to support a medical countermeasure acquisition under Project BioShield using the Special Reserve Fund (see Project BioShield).
Medical Consequence Assessment (MCA)	A process of evaluating the physiological effects for the affected population of a real or hypothetical incident or event that results in injury, illness, or loss of life. This process incorporates individual or group judgment of available information, which may include the quantitative results of medical consequence models.
Medical Counter-measures (MCMs)	Medical countermeasures include both pharmaceutical interventions, such as vaccines, antimicrobials, antidotes, and antitoxins, and non-pharmaceutical interventions, such as ventilators, diagnostics, personal protective equipment (PPE), and patient decontamination that may be used to prevent, mitigate, or treat the adverse health effects of an intentional, accidental, or naturally occurring public health emergency.
Pandemic and All- Hazards Preparedness Act (PAHPA)	Passed by Congress in December 2006 "to improve the Nation's public health and medical preparedness and response capabilities for emergencies, whether deliberate, accidental, or natural." PAHPA amends the Public Health Service Act to require the Secretary of HHS to lead all Federal public health and medical response to public health emergencies and incidents covered by the (former) National Response

(Continued)

	Plan, or what is now the National Response Framework. Among its provisions, the Act established ASPR and provided authorities for a number of programs, including the advanced development and acquisition of medical countermeasures, and called for the establishment of a quadrennial National Health Security Strategy.
HHS Public Health Emergency Medical Counter-measures Enterprise (PHEMCE)	The PHEMCE was established by HHS in 2006 to coordinate Federal efforts to enhance CBRN and EID preparedness from a medical countermeasure perspective. The PHEMCE's mission is to advance national preparedness for CBRN and EID threats, including pandemic influenza, by coordinating medical countermeasure-related efforts within HHS and in cooperation with PHEMCE partners. The PHEMCE is led by the ASPR and includes three core HHS agency partners: CDC, FDA, and NIH. The PHEMCE also includes four interagency partners: DHS, DoD, VA, and USDA. PHEMCE agencies work to protect the American public from national health security threats through the use of medical countermeasures.
Public Health Response Assessment	A process of evaluating the public health response to a real or hypothetical incident or event by explicitly considering concepts of operations. This process incorporates individual or group judgment of available information, which may include the quantitative results of public health response models.
Point of Dispensing (POD)	A designated location for rapidly distributing medical countermeasures, usually antibiotics or vaccines, to high volumes of exposed and potentially exposed persons in a public health emergency. PODs represent the traditional mass prophylaxis distribution method and are not designed to deliver medical care.
PROJECT BIOSHIELD	Signed into law on July 21, 2004, the Project BioShield Act of 2004 represents part of a broader strategy to defend America against the threat of weapons of mass destruction. Project BioShield approaches this goal in three ways: • **Funding of Needed Countermeasures**: Project BioShield institutes a secure funding source and procedures for the purchase of critical medical countermeasures, such as vaccines, therapeutics, and diagnostics, targeted at threats for which an MTD has been issued by DHS (see MTDs). Project BioShield authorizes $5.6 billion in funding through 2013 for the advanced development and purchase of priority medical countermeasures. Acquisitions using this "Special Reserve Fund" are managed by BARDA. • **Facilitating Research and Development**: Project BioShield grants the NIH/National Institute of Allergy and Infectious Diseases authorities to expedite and simplify the solicitation, review, and award of grants and contracts for the development of critical medical countermeasures. • **Facilitating the Use of Medical Countermeasures in an Emergency**: Project BioShield establishes the EUA mechanism to

	provide access to the best available medical countermeasures following the determination of an emergency by the Secretary of DoD, DHS, or HHS, a declaration justifying the EUA by the Secretary of HHS, and issuance of the EUA by the FDA Commissioner.
Recovery	Those capabilities necessary to assist communities affected by an incident to recover effectively, including but not limited to, rebuilding infrastructure systems; providing adequate interim and long-term housing for survivors; restoring health, social, and community services; promoting economic development; and restoring natural and cultural resources.
Response	Immediate actions to save lives, protect property and the environment, and meet basic human needs. Response also includes the execution of emergency plans and actions to support short-term recovery.
Risk	Potential for an adverse outcome assessed as a function of threats (likelihood), vulnerabilities, and consequences associated with an incident, event, or occurrence.
Risk Assessment (RA)	Product or process which collects information and assigns values to risks for the purpose of informing priorities, developing or comparing courses of action, and informing decision making.
Scenario	Hypothetical situation consisting of a hazard, an entity impacted by that hazard, and associated conditions including consequences when appropriate.
Strategic National Stockpile (SNS)	The statutory mission of the SNS is to provide for the emergency health security of the United States (42 USC 247d-6b(a)). The SNS is the Federal cache of pharmaceuticals, vaccines, medical supplies, equipment, and other items established to augment local supplies of critical medical countermeasures that may be needed for a public health emergency or disaster. The SNS is managed by the CDC and includes (1) the 12-Hour Push Packages positioned in strategically located, secure warehouses ready for immediate deployment to a designated site within 12 hours of the federal decision to deploy SNS assets, (2) SNS-managed inventory, and (3) vendor-managed inventory (to increase efficiency and reduce cost of stockpiling). SNS holdings are supplied to state and local jurisdictions at their request upon federal authorization. Formerly known as the National Pharmaceutical Stockpile (NPS).
Terrorism Risk Assessment	Comprehensive, quantitative assessment of terrorism risk within specified threat type (i.e., C-B-R-N) to inform investments; aid in identifying threats, vulnerabilities, and knowledge gaps; and support strategic risk management planning. DHS S&T conducts four formal terrorism risk assessments: • Biological Terrorism Risk Assessment (BTRA) • Chemical Terrorism Risk Assessment (CTRA) • Integrated Terrorism Risk Assessment (ITRA) • Radiological/Nuclear Terrorism Risk Assessment (RNTRA)

(Continued)

Threat Assessment	Product or process of identifying or evaluating entities, actions, or occurrences, whether natural or man-made, that has or indicates the potential to harm life, information, operations, and/or property.

APPENDIX 2 - ACRONYMS

Acronym	Definition
ARS/ DEARE	Acute Radiation Syndrome and the Delayed Effects of Acute Radiation Exposure
ASPR	Assistant Secretary for Preparedness and Response
BARDA	Biomedical Advanced Research and Development Authority
CBRN	chemical, biological, radiological and nuclear
CDC	Centers for Disease Control and Prevention
CRI	Cities Readiness Initiative
DHS	Department of Homeland Security
DoD	U.S. Department of Defense
DTPA	Diethylenetriamine-pentaacetate
EEC	Enterprise Executive Committee
EID	Emerging infectious disease
ESC	Enterprise Senior Council
EUA	Emergency Use Authorization
FDA	Food and Drug Administration
HHS	U.S. Department of Health and Human Services
IPR	In-process-review
IPTs	Integrated Program Teams
JRO	Joint Requirements Office
MCMi	Medical Countermeasure Initiative
MTD	Material threat determination
NBSB	National Biodefense Science Board
NIAID	National Institute of Allergy and Infectious Diseases
NIH	National Institutes of Health
ODATSD (CBD)	Office of the Deputy Assistant to the Secretary of Defense for Chemical and Biological Defense
PAC	Integrated Portfolio Advisory Committee
PCT	Project coordination teams
PEP	Post-exposure prophylaxis
PHEMCE	Public Health Emergency Medical Countermeasures Enterprise

Acronym	Definition
PPE	Personal protective equipment
PREP	Public Readiness and Emergency Preparedness
SLTT	State, local tribal and territorial
SNS	Strategic National Stockpile
SRF	Special Reserve Fund
TAR	Technical assistance reviews
USDA	U.S. Department of Agriculture
USPS	U.S. Postal Service
VA	U.S. Department of Veterans Affairs
VRBPAC	Vaccines and Related Biological Products Advisory Committee
WG	Working group

APPENDIX 3 – PHEMCE ORGANIZATIONAL STRUCTURE

In July 2006, HHS established the Public Health Emergency Medical Countermeasures Enterprise (PHEMCE or Enterprise). The PHEMCE's mission is to advance national preparedness against chemical, biological, radiological, and nuclear (CBRN) and emerging infectious disease (EID) threats, including pandemic influenza, by coordinating medical countermeasure related efforts within HHS and in cooperation with interagency PHEMCE partners. The forum for cooperation and overall mission fulfillment is the Enterprise Senior Council and its supporting infrastructure (Figure 1). Structurally, the ESC is led by the ASPR and comprised of the senior leadership of NIAID, CDC, and FDA with comparable senior level representatives from DoD, DHS, VA, and USDA. Additional HHS components including the Office of the General Counsel, Office of the Assistant Secretary for Health, Office of the Assistant Secretary for Legislation, and the Office of the Assistant Secretary for Planning and Evaluation participate in a non-voting capacity. The PHEMCE activities are organized and governed using the hierarchy shown in this figure.

Enterprise Senior Council (ESC) – It is the mission of the ESC to provide, on behalf of the HHS Secretary, coordinated, strategic direction and policy oversight for HHS "end-to-end" medical countermeasure preparedness activities, defined as requirements generation, research, early- and late-stage product development, procurement, and utilization planning activities for all threats including CBRN, pandemic influenza, and EID. The ESC is a consensus interagency body chaired by the HHS ASPR, as the HHS Secretary's principal advisor on federal public health and medical preparedness and response for public health emergencies. The HHS principal members are the Director for the Centers for Disease Control and Prevention (CDC), the Director of the National Institute of Allergy and Infectious Diseases (NIAID) within the National Institutes of Health (NIH), and the Commissioner of the Food and Drug Administration (FDA). The principal interagency members are the Assistant Secretary of Defense for Nuclear, Chemical, and Biological Defense Programs, Office of the Under Secretary of Defense for Acquisition, Technology and Logistics from DoD; the Assistant Secretary for Health Affairs and Chief Medical Officer from DHS; the Assistant Secretary for Operations, Security and Preparedness from VA; and the Undersecretary for Food Safety from USDA. As the most senior level in the PHEMCE structure, this group approves major policies, product requirements, and large-scale procurement actions. It also oversees strategic reviews of the activities in each of the major threat portfolios (e.g., anthrax, smallpox, rad/nuc) and is the final reporting body for high priority actions identified as gaps in these reviews.

Enterprise Executive Committee (EEC) – The EEC is an operational-level decision and coordination body for all policy and product-level issues in the Enterprise. The EEC is comprised of senior program managers across the partner agencies. It provides the critical interface and organizing capability between the strategic focus of the ESC and the tactical-level efforts conducted within the subordinate Integrated Program Teams (IPTs) and Working Groups (WGs). The EEC reports directly to, and receives guidance from, the ESC. The Executive Committee is co-chaired by two senior management officials appointed by the ASPR. The EEC is composed of senior staff from each PHEMCE agency selected by the ESC members. The EEC is responsible for assuring that important programmatic, procurement, requirements, and portfolio actions are fully vetted and that the solutions and recommended actions requiring approval at higher levels are well delineated for decisions. Additionally, the EEC manages the work at the lower IPT and subgroup levels, directly manages the annual assessment of the Strategic National Stockpile, and composes PHEMCE level documents, such as this Strategy and Implementation Plan.

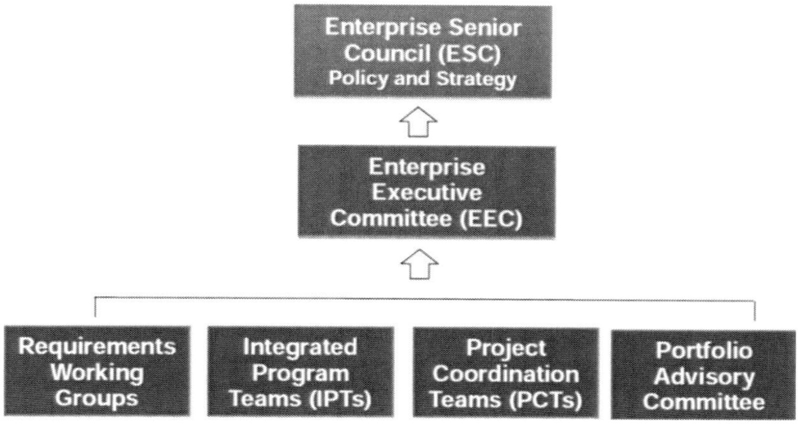

Figure 1. PHEMCE Governance Structure.

Integrated Program Teams (IPTs) – The IPTs provide an end-to-end vision of medical countermeasures against a particular threat type (e.g., anthrax, smallpox) or capability (e.g., diagnostics) that ranges from requirements-setting (specifically quantity and product characteristics) through to stockpiling, delivery and dispensing, and monitoring and evaluating medical countermeasure effectiveness. The IPTs develop strategies for addressing key cross- cutting issues, in consideration of available programmatic resources at the Federal, state, local, tribal and territorial levels. IPTs serve as subject matter expert communities of practice for interagency vetting and input on issues within their purview. They report to the EEC.

Requirements Working Groups (WGs) – The Biological, Chemical, Radiological/Nuclear, and Blood/Tissue MCM Requirements Working Groups are established by the EEC to determine which types of medical countermeasures, including blood and tissue, are needed for response to public health emergencies and other threats to national health security. The Working Groups report to the EEC.

Project Coordination Teams (PCTs) – PCTs are established by the BARDA Director to support the development and administration of each medical countermeasure acquisition or advanced development program managed by BARDA.

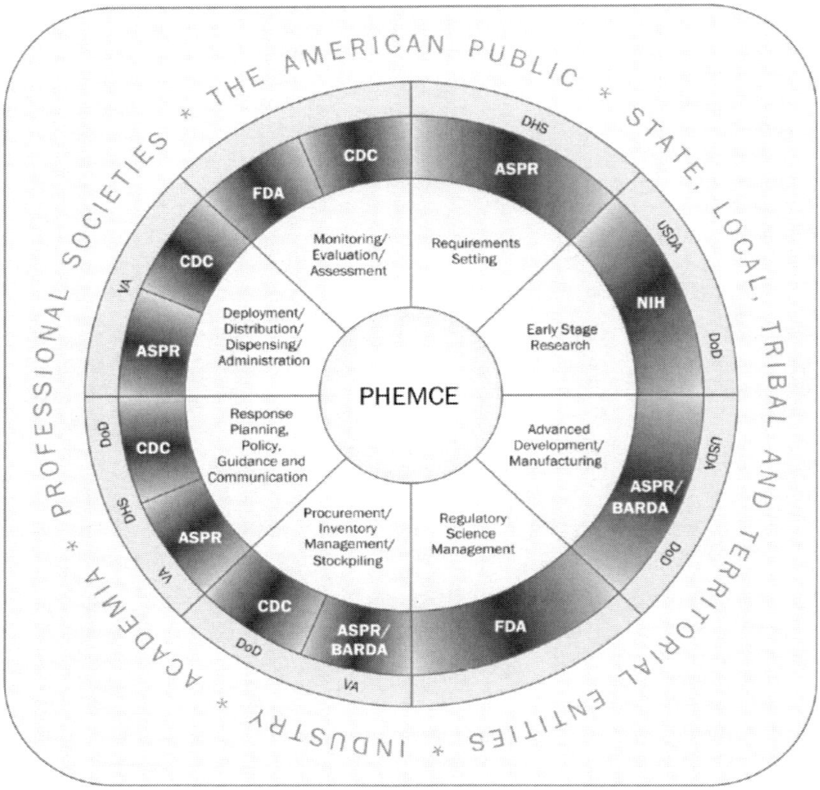

Key:

PHEMCE Mission Components HHS PHEMCE Agencies

Non-HHS PHEMCE Agencies Non-Federal Stakeholders

Acronyms:

PHEMCE: Public Health Emergency Medical Countermeasure Enterprise
DHS: Department of Homeland Security **DoD**: Department of Defense
USDA: U.S. Department of Agriculture **VA**: Department of Veterans' Affairs
HHS: Department of Health and Human Services
ASPR: Assistant Secretary for Preparedness and Response
BARDA: Biomedical Advanced Research & Development Authority
CDC: Centers for Disease Control and Prevention
FDA: Food and Drug Administration **NIH**: National Institutes of Health

Figure 2. PHEMCE Agency Lead Roles.

Integrated Portfolio for CBRN Medical Countermeasures/Portfolio Advisory Committee (PAC) – The PAC seeks to maximize national preparedness to respond to CBRN threats by aligning HHS and DoD MCM development and related infrastructure resources. The PAC reports to the EEC. The activities of the PAC enhance intra- and inter-departmental collaboration in CBRN MCM development, establish a shared understanding of each agency's programmatic requirements, and develop an integrated set of goals. The PAC is co-chaired by the BARDA Principal Deputy Director and by the Medical Director of the Office of the Deputy Assistant to the Secretary of Defense for Chemical and Biological Defense (ODATSD(CBD)).

Specific PHEMCE mission components – and organizations with lead responsibilities and capabilities in these areas – are depicted below (Figure 2).[23] This figure shows the complex interconnectedness of the PHEMCE organizations and mission space.

APPENDIX 4 – PROGRESS REPORT

MCM Program	2007 PHEMCE Implementation Plan Goals[24]	HHS Accomplishments Since 2007
Diagnostics	Development and acquisition of *in vitro* diagnostics for biological agents	• Senior level interagency groups, to include a PHEMCE IPT, have been established to coordinate and leverage the development of specific requirements and diagnostic tools for biothreat diagnostics and ensure integration with the national architecture for the Laboratory Response Network and related networks.
Broad spectrum antibiotic(s)	Evaluation of SNS-held antibiotics and acquisition of commercially available antibiotics as needed; advanced development of broad spectrum antimicrobials addressing bacterial agent material threat determinations (MTDs), including regulatory approval	• BARDA established advanced development programs for new broad-spectrum antibiotics to address both biodefense and routine indications. • NIH developed and FDA accepted a new animal model to support licensure of currently stockpiled antibiotics for use against pneumonic plague. • NIH developed and submitted for FDA review efficacy data to support additional indications for currently available antibiotics. • FDA reviewed and processed several "pre-Emergency Use Authorization

(Continued)

MCM Program	2007 PHEMCE Implementation Plan Goals[24]	HHS Accomplishments Since 2007
	for biodefense clinical indications	(EUA)" submissions for the use of antimicrobial products for first responders and affected populations as part of critical emergency preparedness activities for the 2008 Political Conventions and the 2009 Presidential Inauguration. • An EUA was issued in July 2011 for the emergency use of oral doxycycline for the post-exposure prophylaxis (PEP) of inhalational anthrax. This EUA remains in effect as of this writing. • An EUA was issued for the emergency use of doxycycline hyclate tablet emergency kits for PEP of inhalational anthrax for United States Postal Service (USPS) participants and their household members aspart of the Cities Readiness Initiative (CRI) in October 2008. This EUA was revised in Feb 2009 and October 2011 and remains in effect as of this writing. • CDC conducts ongoing procurement of broad spectrum antibiotics to maintain inventory levels at, or above, PHEMCE requirements.
Broad Spectrum Antivirals	Prioritization of research and development of MCMs capable of addressing several MTD viruses	• BARDA is supporting development of two smallpox antivirals, one of which may also have routine public health applications for other double-stranded DNA viruses.
Anthrax Antitoxin(s)	Continue advanced development and phased acquisition program.	• NIH developed four anthrax antitoxin products through Phase I clinical trials with transition to BARDA for further advanced development. • BARDA supports advanced development of both monoclonal and polyclonal products and development of products with the potential for extended shelf-life, increased ease of administration, and decreased life cycle management cost. • BARDA acquired anthrax antitoxin (of two different types) for the SNS and the

MCM Program	2007 PHEMCE Implementation Plan Goals[24]	HHS Accomplishments Since 2007
		majority has been delivered to the SNS for potential use under EUA. • Anthrax antitoxin developed through NIH and BARDA efforts and now held in the SNS has already been used to treat patients with naturally-acquired pulmonary anthrax in the both the U.S. and Scotland.
Anthrax Vaccine	Advanced development and acquisition of current and next generation anthrax vaccines	• Promising candidates for improved anthrax vaccines that could greatly increase the amount of vaccine ready for use moved from the research bench at NIH to advanced development at BARDA. • NIH completed anthrax vaccine post-exposure prophylaxis (PEP) animal model efficacy development, including (in conjunction with FDA and CDC) utilization of a regulatory pathway validated by FDA's VRBPAC.[25] • BARDA supports advanced development of next generation anthrax vaccines, as well as enhance-ments to the current licensed vaccine and expansion of domestic manufacturing capacity for this product. • HHS acquired the currently licensed anthrax vaccine for the SNS and CDC maintains a contract to support delivery (through 2015) at the maximum levels available within current production capacity to build the SNS holdings towards the existing PHEMCE requirement. • HHS and DoD have consolidated management of their once separate anthrax vaccine stockpiles through the SNS, thus reducing costs and improving the life-cycle management of these vaccines.
Filovirus MCM(s)[26]	Research and development and acquisition of antivirals and/or vaccines	• NIH is funding early stage research in this area

(Continued)

MCM Program	2007 PHEMCE Implementation Plan Goals[24]	HHS Accomplishments Since 2007
Smallpox Antiviral(s)	Advanced development and acquisition	• NIH developed two smallpox antiviral candidates through Phase I and II, respectively, with transition to BARDA for further advanced development and acquisition. • BARDA is funding advanced research and development in this area (see also Broad Spectrum Antivirals) and has awarded a Project BioShield contract for acquisition of a smallpox antiviral.
Smallpox Vaccine	Advanced development and acquisition	• NIH developed a smallpox vaccine candidate through Phase II with transition to BARDA for further advanced development and acquisition. • BARDA funded advanced development of two smallpox vaccines. • BARDA supported advanced development and acquisition for the SNS of a smallpox vaccine for immuno compromised individuals. • HHS also provides the currently licensed smallpox vaccine to DoD through Economy Act orders.
ARS/DEARE[27] MCM(s)	Research, advanced development, and phased acquisition of ARS/DEARE MCM(s)	• BARDA has supported advanced research and development of over 32 different candidate products to mitigate the negative effects of radiation exposure. These products include MCMs to address radiation exposure injuries to the skin, lung, hematopoietic system, and gastrointestinal tract.
Biodosimetry and Bioassay	Advanced development and acquisition of on-scene triage biodosimetry assays; establishment of a system of laboratories	• BARDA supports advanced research and development of several different promising technologies in this area.
Radionuclide-Specific Agent(s)	Development of novel and improved formulations of decorporating agents;	• BARDA acquired liquid Potassium Iodide (KI) (a blocking agent); delivery to the SNS is completed. • BARDA acquired two forms of DTPA; delivery to the SNS is completed.

MCM Program	2007 PHEMCE Implementation Plan Goals[24]	HHS Accomplishments Since 2007
	acquisition of an oral formulation of DTPA[28]	• BARDA supports advanced development of a new formulation of Prussian blue decorporation agent for use in children and of new formulations of DTPA.
Enterprise CHEMPACKs	Procurement and fielding of additional current CHEMPACK configurations; development of operations analysis to support an Enterprise CHEMPACK system;[29] and development and acquisition of next-generation replacement products	• BARDA supports advanced development of a next-generation anticonvulsant product for CHEMPACKs. • CDC completed fielding of CHEMPACK caches to the 50 states, 4 directly-funded cities, all participating U.S. territories, and freely-associated island nations.
Volatile Nerve Agent Single Antidote	Research and development	• In conjunction with NIH, BARDA supports advanced research and development of MCMs for chemical threats.

APPENDIX 5 – STRATEGIC ALIGNMENT

Goal 1: Identify, create, develop, manufacture, and procure critical medical countermeasures	
PHEMCE Mission Components	Requirements Setting; Early Stage Research; Advanced Development/ Manufacturing; Procurement/Inventory Management/Stockpiling
HHS Strategic Plan	Goal 2: Advance Scientific Knowledge and Innovation, Objective A: Accelerate the process of scientific discovery to improve patient care
Secretary's Strategic Initiatives	Accelerate the Process of Scientific Discovery To Improve Patient Care
National Health Security Strategy	Strategic Objective 6: Promote an effective countermeasures enterprise
Goal 2: Establish and communicate clear regulatory pathways to facilitate medical countermeasure development and use	
PHEMCE Mission Components	Regulatory Science Management
HHS Strategic Plan	Goal 2: Advance Scientific Knowledge and Innovation, Objective C: Invest in the regulatory sciences to improve food and medical product safety

Secretary's Strategic Initiatives	Accelerate the Process of Scientific Discovery To Improve Patient Care
National Health Security Strategy	Strategic Objective 6: Promote an effective countermeasures enterprise
Goal 3: Develop logistics and operational plans for optimized use of medical countermeasures at all levels of response	
PHEMCE Mission Components	Procurement/Inventory Management/Stockpiling; Response Planning, Policy, Guidance, and Communication; Deployment/Distribution/ Dispensing /Administration; Monitoring/Evaluation/Assessment
HHS Strategic Plan	Goal 3: Advance the Health, Safety, and Well-being of the American People, Objective F: Protect Americans' health and safety during emergencies, and foster resilience in response to emergencies
Secretary's Strategic Initiatives	Protect Americans' Health and Safety during Emergencies, and Foster Resilience in Response to Emergencies
National Health Security Strategy	Strategic Objective 6: Promote an effective countermeasures enterprise
Goal 4: Address medical countermeasure gaps for all sectors of the American population	
PHEMCE Mission Components	Requirements Setting; Early Stage Research; Advanced Development/Manufacturing; Regulatory Science Management; Procurement/Inventory Management/ Stockpiling; Response Planning, Policy, Guidance, and Communication; Deployment/Distribution/ Dispensing/ Administration; Monitoring/Evaluation/Assessment
HHS Strategic Plan	Goal 1: Strengthen Health Care, Objective E: Ensure access to quality, culturally competent care for vulnerable populations; Goal 2: Advance Scientific Knowledge and Innovation, Objective A: Accelerate the process of scientific discovery to improve patient care and Objective C:Invest in the regulatory sciences to improve food and medical product safety; Goal 3: Advance the Health, Safety, and Well-being of the American People, Objective F: Protect Americans' health and safety during emergencies, and foster resilience in response to emergencies
Secretary's Strategic Initiatives	Eliminate Health Disparities; Accelerate the Process of Scientific Discovery To Improve Patient Care; Protect Americans' Health and Safety during Emergencies, and Foster Resilience in Response to Emergencies
National Health Security Strategy	Strategic Objective 6: Promote an effective countermeasures enterprise

End Notes

[1] At-risk individuals have needs in one or more of the following functional areas: communication, medical care, maintaining independence, supervision, and transportation. At-risk groups may include children, senior citizens, and pregnant women as well as people who have disabilities, live in institutionalized settings, are from diverse cultures, have limited English

proficiency or are non-English speaking, are transportation disadvantaged, have chronic medical disorders, or have pharmacological dependency. http://www.phe.gov/preparedness/planning/abc/pages/default.aspx

[2] Medical countermeasures include both pharmaceutical interventions, such as vaccines, antimicrobials, antidotes, and antitoxins, and non-pharmaceutical interventions, such as ventilators, diagnostics, personal protective equipment (PPE), and patient decontamination that may be used to prevent, mitigate, or treat the adverse health effects of an intentional, accidental or naturally occurring public health emergency.

[3] Medical countermeasures include qualified countermeasures as defined in section 319F–1(a)(2) of the Public Health Service Act (42 U.S.C. § 247d–6a(a)(2)); qualified pandemic or epidemic products as defined in section 319F–3(i)(7) of the Public Health Service Act (42 U.S.C. § 247d–6d(i)(7))), and security countermeasures as defined in section 319F-2(c)(1)(B) of the Public Health Service Act (42 U.S.C. § 247d–6b(c)(1)(B)).

[4] See section 2801 of the Public Health Services Act (42 U.S.C. 300hh)

[5] These include but are not limited to the National Strategy for Public Health and Medical Preparedness (Homeland Security Presidential Directive-21, October 2007); the National Response Framework (January 2008); the National Health Security Strategy (December 2009); and the National Preparedness Goal (Presidential Policy Directive – 8, March 2011).

[6] Available at http://www.hhs.gov/secretary/about/priorities/priorities.html

[7] Available at http://www.gpo.gov/fdsys/pkg/FR-2006-07-06/pdf/06-6004.pdf

[8] This mandate includes consideration of the particular needs of first responder populations who are placed at particular risk in the course of their duties and critical infrastructure workers. The role of HHS in working with interagency partners to ensure these populations have access to the support they need, including medical countermeasures, is described elsewhere and not detailed here: http://www.phe.gov/Preparedness/planning/cip/Pages/default.aspx http://www.phe.gov/about/OPP/DHSHCP/Pages/default.aspx http://www.phe.gov/preparedness/planning/postal/Pages/default.aspx.

[9] The Office of the ASPR includes component offices with key PHEMCE roles such as the Biomedical Advanced Research and Development Authority (BARDA), Office of Policy and Planning (OPP), and Office of Preparedness and Emergency Operations (OPEO).

[10] Regulatory Science is the science of developing new tools, standards, and approaches to assess the safety, efficacy, quality, and performance of all FDA-regulated products. http://www.fda.gov/ScienceResearch/SpecialTopics/RegulatoryScience/default.htm?utm_campaign=Google2&utm_source=fdaSearch&utm_medium=website&utm_term=regulatoryscience&utm_content=1.

[11] P.L. 108-276; available at http://www.hsdl.org/?view&did=449237

[12] *Public Health Preparedness: 2011 State-by-State Update on Laboratory Capabilities and Response Readiness Planning.*

[13] Including but not limited to: The FDA *Emergency Use Authorization Final Guidance (July 2007);Guidance for Industry Animal Models – Essential Elements to Address Efficacy under the Animal Rule Draft Guidance (January 2009); Guidance for Industry Qualification Process for Drug Development Tools (October 2010).*

[14] Presidential Policy Directive 8 http://www.whitehouse.gov/blog/2011/10/07/ppd-8-announcing-national-preparedness-goal

[15] *The Public Health Emergency Medical Countermeasures Enterprise Review: Transforming the Enterprise to Meet Long-Range National Needs.* August 2010. http://www.phe.gov/preparedness/mcm/enterprisereview/Pages/default.aspx

[16] Enacted December 30, 2005 (P L. 109-148); Available at ftp://ftp.hrsa.gov/countermeasurescomp/Public_Readiness_and_Emergency_Preparedness_Act.pdf

[17] For purposes of this document, the term "approval" refers to FDA-approval, licensure, or clearance under sections 505, 510(k), or 515 of the Federal Food, Drug, and Cosmetic Act or section 351 of the Public Health Service Act.

[18] Relman DA. Bioterrorism – Preparing to Fight the Next War, *NEJM*, 2006, 354 (2): 113-115. In the context of defense against biological threats, a fixed defense is a medical countermeasure intended for use against a specific organism and not useful in scenarios that employ a different organism.

[19] In situations where potentially useful medical countermeasures are available but not yet FDA-approved, licensed, or cleared for the particular use contemplated, FDA has a variety of regulatory mechanisms that can allow for the use of these products, including as part of a clinical trial or as part of an expanded access program or under an emergency use authorization.

[20] http://www.fda.gov/EmergencyPreparedness/MedicalCountermeasures/default.htm

[21] At-risk individuals have needs in one or more of the following functional areas: communication, medical care, maintaining independence, supervision, and transportation. At-risk groups may include children, senior citizens, and pregnant women as well as people who have disabilities, live in institutionalized settings, are from diverse cultures, have limited English proficiency or are non-English speaking, are transportation disadvantaged, have chronic medical disorders, or have pharmacological dependency. http://www.phe.gov/preparedness/planning/abc/pages/default.aspx

[22] The SNS authority specifically requires that the emergency health security of children and other at-risk populations be taken into account in determining which medical countermeasures and supplies are needed for the SNS (Section 319F-2 of the Public Health Services Act (42 USC 247d-6b)).

[23] While capabilities from across the PHEMCE are utilized in many of these areas, the organizations with lead responsibility in particular areas are specifically depicted here.

[24] HHS advanced development and acquisition goals proposed for the time period FY2007-FY2013.

[25] Vaccines and Related Biological Products Advisory Committee

[26] Medical countermeasures.

[27] Acute Radiation Syndrome and the Delayed Effects of Acute Radiation Exposure

[28] Diethylenetriamine-pentaacetate, a chelating agent.

[29] To include education, training, and exercise components and by optimizing the pre-positioning of antidotes.

In: Public Health Emergency …
Editor: Niel A. Harris

ISBN: 978-1-62808-861-8

Chapter 2

PUBLIC HEALTH EMERGENCY MEDICAL COUNTERMEASURES ENTERPRISE (PHEMCE) IMPLEMENTATION PLAN*

U.S. Department of Health and Human Services

EXECUTIVE SUMMARY

The *2012 Public Health Emergency Medical Countermeasures Enterprise (PHEMCE) Implementation Plan* describes the priorities that HHS, in collaboration with its interagency partners, will implement over the next five years to advance the strategic goals and underlying objectives established in the *2012 PHEMCE Strategy*. Priorities are identified along the near- (Fiscal Year [FY] 12-14), mid- (FY15-17), and long-term (FY18 and beyond) timeframes where appropriate. Together, the *2012 PHEMCE Strategy* and *Implementation Plan* provide the blueprint for the PHEMCE to enhance national health security through the procurement and use of life-saving medical countermeasures (MCMs).

As stated in the *Strategy*, the PHEMCE is driven by two core principles: (1) the medical and public health imperative to limit the potential adverse health impacts posed by a variety of threats, and (2) the fiduciary responsibility to maximize the preparedness that can be gained with the

* This is an edited, reformatted and augmented version of a U.S. Department of Health and Human Services publication, dated December 2012.

significant but finite resources available. The *Implementation Plan* lays out a prioritization framework that is consistent with these core principles, and seeks to best manage the difficult choices facing the PHEMCE, in light of fiscal constraints, scientific limitations, and other factors. Using this prioritization framework the *Implementation Plan* identifies priority activities across the various PHEMCE mission areas, including requirement-setting; basic research; discovery and early development; advanced development; regulatory science management; procurement and stockpiling; response planning; distribution and dispensing; and monitoring, evaluation, and assessment programs. These priorities support the goals and objectives in the *Strategy*, and are summarized in Table 1. The *Implementation Plan* provides both a broad-based description of these priority activities, as well as further detail regarding threat-based and capabilities-based approaches.

The Assistant Secretary for Preparedness and Response (ASPR) will establish an internal tracking mechanism to monitor and evaluate the execution of priorities identified in the *2012 PHEMCE Implementation Plan* and report progress regularly to senior leadership and, to the extent feasible in light of national security and proprietary concerns, to external stakeholders. It is anticipated that the *PHEMCE Strategy* and *Implementation Plan* will be reviewed and updated every five years, or more frequently if needed.

What is the PHEMCE?

The *Public Health Emergency Medical Countermeasures Enterprise (PHEMCE)* is an interagency coordinating body led by the HHS Assistant Secretary for Preparedness and Response (ASPR), comprising the Centers for Disease Control and Prevention (CDC), the National Institutes of Health (NIH), the Food and Drug Administration (FDA), and interagency partners at the Departments of Veterans Affairs (VA), Defense (DoD), Homeland Security (DHS), and Agriculture (USDA). It coordinates the development, acquisition, stockpiling, and use of medical products that are needed to effectively respond to a variety of potential high-consequence public health emergencies, whether naturally occurring or intentional.

Table 1. PHEMCE Priorities by Goals and Objectives

Objective	Phemce Priorities
GOAL 1. Identify, create, develop, manufacture, and procure critical medical countermeasures.	

Objective	Phemce Priorities
Objective 1.1Develop a strategic framework to prioritize PHEMCE resources and investments. (Lead: ASPR; Partners: PHEMCE agencies)	• Establish, evolve, and evaluate a prioritization framework
Objective 1.2Utilize consistent approaches for medical consequence and public health response assessments and medical countermeasure requirement setting that include consideration of effective production, storage, deployment, and administration strategies. (Lead: ASPR; Partners: PHEMCE agencies)	Enhance the development of clear and rigorous civilian MCM requirements, including capabilities-based requirements
Objective 1.3Ensure a robust and sustainable product pipeline for medical countermeasures that emphasizes multi-functional capabilities (e.g., platform technologies, host-based innovations, broad-spectrum medical countermeasures) rather than stand alone outcomes and includes consideration of viable commercial markets and/or routine public health applicability. (Leads: NIH, ASPR; Partners: DoD, CDC, USDA)	• Invest in basic research, discovery, early and advanced development, and acquisition of current and novel MCMs according to the prioritization framework
Objective 1.4Promote effective domestic and international partnerships with developers and manufacturers and support core services. (Leads: ASPR, NIH; Partners: DoD, CDC, FDA, HHS Office of Global Affairs (OGA))	• Maintain a wide array of product development and support service contracts to provide infrastructure capabilities for MCM development and response • Enter into strategic bilateral and multilateral engagements with international partners to identifyjoint opportunities for product development
GOAL 2. Establish and communicate clear regulatory pathways to facilitate medical countermeasure development and use.	
Objective 2.1 Identify scientific and regulatory issues that challenge medical countermeasure development or use during public health emergencies and coordinate activities among PHEMCE partners to address those challenges. (Lead: FDA; Partners: PHEMCE agencies)	• Enhance product review and approval processes for the highest-priority MCMs • Advance regulatory science to support MCM development and regulatory assessment • Assess the legal, regulatory, and policy environments regarding MCM development, distribution, administration, and use and propose new approaches where necessary

Table 1. (Continued)

Objective	Phemce Priorities
Objective 2.2Assist medical countermeasure developers in working interactively with FDA during product development and regulatory review (Lead: FDA; Partners: NIH, ASPR)	• Clarify regulatory pathways and reduce regulatory barriers for MCM developers • Provide product development core services to MCM developers and manufacturers
GOAL 3. Develop logistics and operational plans for optimized use of medical countermeasures at all levels of response.	
Objective 3.1 Promote innovative approaches to inventory management to enable a sustainable preparedness infrastructure (Lead: CDC; Partners: ASPR, DHS)	• Optimize the Strategic National Stockpile (SNS) • formulary • Cost-effectively manage SNS assets Enhance the long-term sustainability of the SNS
Objective 3.2Develop and communicate medical countermeasure utilization policy, guidance and response strategies, including FDA regulatory frameworks, that are responsive to end-user needs and that are integrated with state, local, tribal, territorial (SLTT) and private sector response plans, and when possible international partners, and that ensure timely, safe, and effective medical countermeasure distribution and utilization. (Leads: ASPR, CDC, Partners: PHEMCE agencies, OGA)	• Strengthen the feedback loop between the end-users and developers of MCMs • Develop MCM policies, clinical use guidelines, and federal response strategies to inform end-user planning • Ensure preparedness in key federal policy and response capabilities Support state, local, tribal, and territorial responseefforts Identify and address barriers to building a sustainable MCM global infrastructure
Objective 3.3Develop and provide medical countermeasure communications, training, and education information to inform all stakeholders. (Leads: CDC, ASPR; Partners: FDA, USDA)	• Develop a comprehensive MCM communication program and multi-year implementation plan • Test the effectiveness of MCM-related public health communication materials Develop and implement a plan to disseminate best practices for establishing and maintaining regional coordination for public health emergencies
Objective 3.4Develop and implement strategies to assess, evaluate, and monitor medical countermeasure safety, performance, and patient compliance during and after a public health emergency response. (Leads: FDA, CDC, ASPR)	• Develop an Action Plan that will serve as the overall PHEMCE plan for monitoring the safety and clinical benefit of MCMs during public health emergencies

Objective	Phemce Priorities
GOAL 4. Address medical countermeasure gaps for all sectors of the American civilian population.	
Objective 4.1 Develop medical consequence and public health response assessments and requirements setting for at-risk individuals. (Lead: ASPR; Partners: PHEMCE agencies)	• Consider at-risk population needs in every stage of the MCM requirement-setting process • Support research to close important knowledge gaps regarding susceptibility differences and/or altered disease severity in at-risk populations • Incorporate subject matter expertise to inform the development of MCM requirements and response strategies to ensure availability of safe and effective MCMs for at-risk populations
Objective 4.2 Support medical countermeasure advanced development and procurement for at-risk individuals. (Leads: ASPR, NIH, FDA; Partner: CDC)	• Include consideration of at-risk population needs in SNS formulary analyses • Support expanding MCM label indications to at-risk populations during the development of priorityMCMs, including development of alternate formulations as needed • Leverage existing at-risk population databases fordrugs approved for other indications to demonstrate efficacy for biodefense applications in these populations without the need for additional studies
Objective 4.3 Develop and implement strategies, policies, and guidance to support the appropriate use of medical countermeasures in all civilian populations during an emergency. (Leads: ASPR, CDC; Partner: FDA)	• Address regulatory challenges associated with use of products intended for at-risk populations • Ensure that public health and medical information is delivered in a manner that takes into account the range of communication and other functional • needs of the intended recipients, including at-risk individuals • Identify and comprehensively integrate departmental activities related to the needs of children • Anticipate and proactively address the needs of at-risk populations during a disaster

INTRODUCTION

The *Department of Health and Human Services (HHS) 2012 Public Health Emergency Medical Countermeasures Enterprise (PHEMCE) Strategy*[1] (Strategy) defined the strategic goals and objectives to provide the nation with a nimble, flexible capability to rapidly produce and effectively utilize medical countermeasures (MCMs) in the face of any attack or threat, whether known or unknown, novel or reemerging, natural, accidental, or intentional. The HHS *2012 PHEMCE Implementation Plan* (Implementation Plan) details those HHS programs and initiatives from across the PHEMCE mission components[2] that will be pursued to achieve the goals and objectives established in the Strategy. The Implementation Plan thus updates and builds upon the initial efforts contained in the *2007 PHEMCE Strategy* and *Implementation Plan.*[3] The 2012 Strategy and Implementation Plan also support and complement the *2009 National Health Security Strategy (NHSS)*[4] and the *2012 NHSS Implementation Plan*[5] (particularly Strategic Objective 6, which calls for promotion of an effective countermeasure enterprise).

As detailed in the 2012 PHEMCE Strategy, the PHEMCE is an interagency coordinating body led by the HHS Assistant Secretary for Preparedness and Response (ASPR), comprising the Centers for Disease Control and Prevention (CDC), the National Institutes of Health (NIH), the Food and Drug Administration (FDA), and interagency partners at the Departments of Veterans Affairs (VA), Defense (DoD), Homeland Security (DHS), and Agriculture (USDA). The PHEMCE coordinates the development, acquisition, stockpiling, and use of medical products that are needed to respond to a variety of potential high-consequence public health emergencies.

The Implementation Plan has four primary sections: (1) A high-level description of the programs and initiatives that will be pursued by HHS, in coordination with its interagency partners, to accomplish each goal and objective described in the Strategy; (2) an overview of PHEMCE interagency partner roles and collaborations; (3) a detailed description of priorities organized by threat(s); and (4) a description of specific activities addressing multiple needs and/or threats – also known as capability-based approaches. Plans to pursue and accomplish all priority activities and initiatives detailed in this Plan are based upon currently anticipated funding levels over the five-year lifetime of the Plan.

ASPR will monitor and evaluate the execution of priorities identified in the plan and report progress regularly to senior leadership. Throughout the document, each initiative is preceded by an activity code to facilitate subsequent tracking. A subset of key implementation plan milestones in the near and mid-terms is summarized in Appendix 2.

SECTION 1: ACTIVITIES TO ACHIEVE STRATEGIC GOALS AND OBJECTIVES

The Strategy presented four major goals, aligned to capture: (1) the overall prioritization of PHEMCE resources and MCM development and procurement activities; (2) regulatory enhancements to facilitate MCM development and use; (3) logistical and operational plans for optimal MCM use in a public health emergency; and (4) consideration of at-risk population MCM needs. This section describes the broad programs and initiatives that HHS, in collaboration with its interagency partners, will implement over the next five years to advance the strategic goals and underlying objectives called out in the Strategy. Where appropriate, lead and partner agencies are called out, and activities are projected for near- (FY12-14), mid- (FY15-17) and long-range (FY18 and beyond) timeframes. More detailed information on these priorities is provided in Sections 3 and 4 of this report, organized by specific threat area and cross-cutting technologies or approaches, respectively.

Goal 1. Identify, create, develop, manufacture, and procure critical medical countermeasures.

Objective 1.1. Develop a strategic framework to prioritize PHEMCE resources and investments. (*Lead: ASPR; Partners: PHEMCE agencies)*

PHEMCE Prioritization Framework: Principles and Criteria

Prior to the development of this document, various efforts to support strategic prioritization were_already ongoing across the PHEMCE. During the development of this plan, the PHEMCE initiated an effort to explicitly articulate the common prioritization framework underlying past and present PHEMCE strategic decisions. This newly articulated framework, presented here, served as the foundation for selecting the priority programs and initiatives described in this Implementation Plan, and will form the basis for key strategic decisions moving forward.

Core Principles

1. Medical and public health imperative to limit the adverse health impacts posed by a variety of threats
2. Fiscal responsibility to be prudent with resources entrusted to the PHEMCE

The PHEMCE prioritization framework is based on the two core principles that lay the foundation for PHEMCE priorities, as detailed in the Strategy: (1) the medical and public health imperative to limit the potential adverse health impacts posed by a variety of threats, and (2) the fiduciary responsibility to be prudent with the significant but limited resources entrusted to the programs by Congress and the nation while maximizing preparedness. The PHEMCE prioritization framework represents these core principles, and uses three primary and three moderating criteria for identifying priority investments, as described below.

The primary criteria are:

- Threat: The PHEMCE will pursue appropriate investments against high-priority threats6 for which sufficient MCM capabilities do not exist, and focus resources in those areas that pose the greatest threat to national health security. These include chemical, biological, radiological, and nuclear (CBRN) threats, as well as naturally occurring ones such as pandemic influenza and other emerging infectious diseases. The PHEMCE leadership determination as to which of these pose the greatest threats is informed by current levels of MCM preparedness, intelligence information and risk assessments, the evolution of adversary capabilities, scientific advances, and patterns of newly emerging or reemerging infectious diseases.
- Multi-Functionality: The PHEMCE will prioritize investments for those programs and initiatives that may provide agile capabilities suitable for a wide range of known and unknown threats, including products with routine public health applicability. This includes maximizing the potential for broad-spectrum applicability against multiple threats (including adaptable expression and manufacturing platforms), leveraging viable commercial markets, and developing

manufacturing flexibility. The intent is to move, where possible, from narrow applications and approaches to those with broader applicability, with the goal of improving cost-effectiveness while enhancing response flexibility.

- Operational Capacity: A major factor in prioritization is the degree to which a product is operationally and logistically practical and acceptable to its end-users.7 This includes a focus on adapting MCM distribution and use methods to take advantage of "everyday" systems to the greatest extent possible. Current and future product improvements will focus on aspects such as ease of administration,8 simplified shipping and storage, routine use in healthcare,9 and regulatory status,10 all of which are key considerations in assessing the ability to effectively utilize a particular MCM in an emergency.

Primary Criteria

1. Threat Priority
2. Multi-Functionality
3. Operational Capacity

Moderating Criteria

1. At risk-Population Needs
2. Time to Product Availability
3. Lifecycle Cost

The moderating criteria are:

- At-Risk Population Needs: The PHEMCE will continue to strive to address the needs of all segments of the U.S. civilian population, including at-risk populations. While there are difficult technical and cost considerations inherent in the development of MCMs that would address the needs of each at-risk population,11 the PHEMCE will consider all alternatives, including development of alternative formulations and delivery routes, or other suitable operational solutions that can help ensure that the needs of at-risk populations are addressed.
- Time: The time to access MCMs currently in the development process will be considered when allocating resources across PHEMCE

portfolios. Whenever possible in considering alternative products to pursue, the PHEMCE will seek a balance between the most rapid returns on investment, and significant gains in capabilities that may be possible through longer sustained efforts. Investments will be structured to ensure a sufficient level of preparedness today, while pursuing transformational achievements that could promise even greater preparedness enhancements in the future.

- Cost: The lifecycle costs of MCMs will be considered holistically, including development, acquisition, and long-term sustainment needs.

PHEMCE Prioritization Processes and Activities

The PHEMCE has taken significant steps toward developing methods to prioritize resource allocations for MCM development and response needs. Key elements of such prioritization processes have already been embodied in the strengthened governance structure for the PHEMCE (detailed in the Strategy) developed in response to the *2010 PHEMCE Review.*[12] This next phase of PHEMCE management will see an evolution of these methods. Primary activities to implement the prioritization framework will include:

- (1.1.1) Strategic End-States (near-term): By the end of FY13, ASPR will lead PHEMCE agencies to define strategic end-states for all PHEMCE capabilities based on a clear description of the preparedness goals for addressing particular threats and/or MCM needs. Targets for specific MCM levels and types, along with well-delineated operational capabilities to distribute and assess impact, are essential elements of a decision process for prioritizing across PHEMCE domains.
- (1.1.2) Portfolio Reviews (ongoing): ASPR leads the periodic (at least every 18 months) review of specific MCM portfolios across the PHEMCE to monitor progress in MCM preparedness, identify remaining gaps and challenges, and develop potential solutions. These Portfolio Reviews will continue providing a venue to foster coordination among PHEMCE partner agencies in the identification of those areas requiring additional attention and resource prioritization.
- (1.1.3) Multi-Year Budgeting (ongoing): Development of the multi-year budgeting initiative, called for in the 2010 PHEMCE Review,

was initiated in 2011 and this budgeting tool has continued to evolve since then. It will be used in the future to more tightly link investments across NIH, ASPR, CDC, and FDA. This process will help to drive projection of future budget needs within and among agencies as MCM products mature and move across agency boundaries in the development and procurement processes.

- (1.1.4) Portfolio Management (near-term): ASPR will implement PHEMCE-wide portfolio tracking tools by the end of FY13 to further enable coordinated planning and management of CBRN MCM development. (1.1.5) The PHEMCE will consider expansion of the portfolio tracking tools to include pandemic influenza or other Emerging Infectious Diseases (EID) portfolios as needed by FY18. These tools will provide a common set of business practices and harmonized performance metrics that will facilitate benchmarking and data-driven management practices to achieve shorter timelines and greater cost-efficiencies in MCM development portfolios. Furthermore, these tools will be incorporated into an annual strategic portfolio-wide management assessment review incorporating state-of-the-art methods that will help readjust resource allocations to programs that demonstrate acceptable returns on investment.
- (1.1.6)Decision Tools (ongoing): The PHEMCE will develop systematic approaches to decision-making within particular PHEMCE mission areas. For example, to support the PHEMCE's Strategic National Stockpile (SNS) Annual Review process,13 discussed in greater detail under Objective 3.1 below, the PHEMCE has developed a decision support tool, the Relative Priority Index (RPI). The RPI brings the PHEMCE prioritization framework criteria to bear in evaluating the SNS holdings.

Over the next five years, the PHEMCE prioritization framework will be further developed, implemented, and evaluated. *(1.1.7)* Development activities will focus over the next year on the improvement of a suite of analytic decision support and visualization tools and models. *(1.1.8)* Implementation activities will then focus on enhancing the decision-making process by which PHEMCE leadership prioritizes resource allocations. *(1.1.9)* Evaluation activities conducted in the mid term will assess strengths and limitations of the framework components. This approach will allow for a consistent process to develop best practices that most effectively meet the needs of PHEMCE decision-makers in evaluating investment strategies.

Objective 1.2. Utilize consistent approaches for medical consequence and public health response assessments and medical countermeasure requirement setting that include consideration of effective production, storage, deployment, and administration strategies. (*Lead: ASPR; Partners: PHEMCE agencies)*

The PHEMCE will enhance the development of civilian MCM requirements that detail the types and quantities of critical MCMs that would be needed to address various threats. ASPR, working with public health, technical, and scientific experts across the PHEMCE, leads the development of these requirements and vets them through the PHEMCE governance structure prior to finalization via signature of the ASPR. MCM requirements provide projections of the number of people who could benefit from MCMs, along with desired product characteristics. The requirements thus provide a critical piece of information to support PHEMCE leadership allocation of limited resources. Prior to making investment decisions, however, the PHEMCE considers MCM needs across the entire threat portfolio, along with scientific opportunity, available resources, and other factors, using the PHEMCE prioritization framework described previously.

A number of key factors will be considered in developing these enhanced requirements. These include:

- *Threat and risk assessments and PHEMCE-approved planning scenarios*: DHS leads the development of Terrorism Risk Assessments (TRAs),[14] Material Threat Assessments (MTAs),[15] and Material Threat Determinations (MTDs),[16] with support from other PHEMCE partner agencies. These documents identify the scale and nature of potential threats, which then inform HHS modeling of the estimated public health impact and response needs. *(1.2.1)* Over the next year, HHS, DHS, and other agencies (e.g., the Environmental Protection Agency, Department of Justice, and Office of the Director of National Intelligence) will work to formalize roles, responsibilities, policies, and procedures for conducting the next generation of MTAs and TRAs. These collaborations, along with close coordination with the intelligence community, will ensure that PHEMCE requirements for intentional threats are based on the most accurate threat information available. This effort should result in an integrated process that provides a sound, science-based analytic foundation for the PHEMCE to define and prioritize MCM requirements and planning. Next-generation MTAs and TRAs will support decisions by DHS, HHS, and other agency leadership; improve PHEMCE MCM requirements; and inform threat awareness and biodefense-related investments to support emergency preparedness, planning, and response efforts. The ESC will also request that MCM requirement-setting and planning be conducted for those naturally occurring and accidental threats to national health security that are outside the realm of the DHS threat and risk assessments.

- *Public health response and medical consequence assessments:* The Biomedical Advanced Research and Development Authority (BARDA), within ASPR,[17] develops scenario-based medical consequence and public health response models as key inputs to the generation of civilian MCM requirements. CDC conducts specialized public health modeling to predict disease emergence, disease spread, and outbreak response. *(1.2.2)* BARDA will augment current models and will work with the CDC over the next two years to develop updated disease assessments based on refinements of available data sources and modeling methodologies.
- *CONOPs considerations*: Consideration of the current and anticipated Concepts of Operations (CONOPs) and public health response capabilities at the federal and state, local, tribal, and territorial (SLTT) levels is critical to ensure that stockpiled MCMs can be safely and effectively used in a public health emergency. PHEMCE requirements are based on MCM deployment strategies and utilization policies supported by present and future programmed federal and SLTT capabilities to rapidly ship, distribute, and dispense these products. For example, CDC has developed several modeling tools that facilitate planning at the federal and SLTT levels, providing officials with ways to evaluate plans without resource-intensive drills or exercises. CDC also has developed epidemiologic modeling tools that can be used in response to a public health emergency, such as a pandemic influenza outbreak, to inform MCM utilization policy, clinical guidance, and response strategies.[18] *(1.2.3)* In the mid term, CDC will enhance its modeling capability and collaborations in order to better determine the burden of disease and effect of interventions.

(1.2.4) In the near term, ASPR, working with subject matter experts from across the PHEMCE, will develop or update specific MCM requirements to address:

- Biological threats
  - *Anthrax* – including harmonization of planning scenarios underlying all anthrax MCM requirements, as well as specific requirements for diagnostics, vaccines, and antitoxins for treatment
  - *Botulism* – including antitoxins for treatment
  - *Glanders and meliodosis*
- Chemical threats – including requirements for cyanide antidotes, acetylcholinesterase reactivators, and neuroprotectants, as well as MCM needs for vesicant and pulmonary agents and patient decontamination
- Nuclear threats – including requirements for addressing the components of acute radiation syndrome, pulmonary radiation injury, antimicrobial needs, anti-emetics, biodosimetry, and other MCM needs
- Radiological threats – including requirements for addressing bioassay diagnostics and MCMs for internalized radioisotopes prioritized through the PHEMCE
- Multiple threats
  - Thermal burn products
  - Ventilators
  - Blood products – including requirements for MCMs targeting thrombocytopenia and lymphopenia, as well as for blood substitutes and aplastic reconstitutors

(1.2.5) In the mid term, ASPR will develop or update the MCM requirements for:

- Biological threats
  - Anthrax – including more detailed requirements for point-of-care and multiplex anthrax diagnostics
  - Broad-spectrum antimicrobials – including requirements for both treatment and prophylaxis
  - Filovirus – including requirements for diagnostics, prophylaxis, and treatment

    - Smallpox – including requirements for Vaccinia Immune Globulin (VIG) to treat complications from smallpox vaccination
- Chemical threats – including requirements for diagnostics and MCMs to address the effects of GABA antagonists
- Nuclear threats – including requirements for products to address the effects of radiation exposure on the kidneys, as well as for utilization of vasopressors and needs for analgesics and anesthetics
- Radiological threats – including more detailed requirements for chelators such as DTPA and other MCMs needed to address these threats

In support of the emphasis being placed by the PHEMCE on fostering more capabilities-based approaches that support multi-functionality, ASPR will also develop capabilities-based requirements that capture MCM needs in broad areas, with a strong emphasis on end-user needs. *(1.2.6)* In the near term (FY12-14), such initial capabilities documents will be developed for biological diagnostics, CBRN therapeutics, prophylaxis for biological threats, and non-pharmaceutical MCM needs such as ventilators and respirators. In addition, as priorities dictate and resources allow, the PHEMCE will continue to develop requirements to address any new threats determined by DHS to pose a material threat to national security. *(1.2.7)* In addition, analytical tools will be developed to demonstrate the effect of fulfilling any particular requirement on overall threat preparedness, in support of strategic decision-making within the PHEMCE prioritization framework.

PHEMCE requirements will continue to be a key factor in informing HHS-supported MCM research, development, and acquisition priorities. This information is publicly communicated to stakeholders, including industry, at the time of advanced research and development or acquisition solicitations. In the long term, all MCM requirements will be revisited periodically to allow incorporation of new threat assessments, MCM technologies, and response capabilities.

Objective 1.3 Ensure a robust and sustainable product pipeline for medical countermeasures that emphasizes multi-functional capabilities (e.g., platform technologies, host-based innovations, broad-spectrum medical countermeasures) rather than stand alone outcomes and includes consideration of viable commercial markets and/or routine public health applicability. (Leads: NIH, ASPR; Partners: DoD, CDC, USDA)

As defined in the 2012 PHEMCE Strategy, MCMs include both pharmaceutical interventions (e.g., vaccines, antimicrobials, antidotes, and antitoxins) and non-pharmaceutical MCM interventions (e.g., ventilators, diagnostics, personal protective equipment, and patient decontamination methods) that may be used to prevent, mitigate, or treat the adverse health effects of a public health emergency. Major investments have been made in these areas since the last PHEMCE Strategy and Implementation Plan were released in 2007, and this Implementation Plan expands the pursuit of these products. Continued investment in current and new technologies will be based on satisfying the prioritization criteria and requirements defined above.

The civilian MCM product pipeline predominantly comprises research and advanced development efforts supported through the combined efforts of NIH and BARDA, in coordination with DoD and CDC, that have direct relevance to civilian national health security. The PHEMCE is at a point of inflection as it moves from addressing near-term needs, often with MCMs that address a single threat, to longer-term, capabilities-based systems with the flexibility to address multiple, known and unknown threats. While this system introduces change where possible to allow for a more flexible, capabilities-based approach, it is essential that current single-threat focused products that are under development or planned for acquisition remain available to address immediate needs. The PHEMCE considers at-risk population needs throughout its efforts to ensure a robust and sustainable product pipeline; activities specifically directed at addressing at-risk population needs will be described in detail under Goal 4 of this section.

(1.3.1) NIH will focus on the basic and translational research, and the expansion of research infrastructure and resources that are the fundamental building blocks for developing civilian MCMs. *(1.3.2)* NIH will also assume responsibility for evaluation of previously licensed, off-patent countermeasures in an effort to expand approved indications to other threat agents or infectious diseases, as well as increase the repertoire of countermeasures with pediatric indications. *(1.3.3)* In addition, NIH will continue to develop and test new products and approaches to treatment and infection control (e.g., multi-component vaccines, broad-spectrum antimicrobials, and point-of-care and broad-spectrum diagnostics).

(1.3.4) Through FY17, NIH will emphasize the early-stage research programs listed in Table 2 (more details on particular programs are provided in

Sections 3 and 4). Early-stage products that demonstrate promise for advanced development will be brought to the attention of BARDA through regular communications and opportunities for technology transfer. *(1.3.5)* For example, over the next five years, multiple candidates for a next-generation anthrax vaccine, broad- spectrum antiviral drug, influenza antiviral drug, and potentially a next-generation influenza vaccine may be available for advanced development consideration.

(1.3.6) NIH will also continue to manage the Concept Acceleration Program (CAP) to create and coordinate teams of scientific, medical, and product development experts to guide investigators working on multi-use products for biodefense, drug resistance, and emerging disease applications. The CAP was initiated as a result of the *2010 PHEMCE Review* to accelerate the development of promising, high-priority MCMs. For example, recently a unique collaboration of NIH and extramural scientists funded by CAP led to identification of a host target for filoviruses that suggests an already licensed drug could be effective against threats such as Ebola virus.[24] Further studies in this area are currently being conducted.

NIH's long-term focus (FY18 and beyond) will increase the emphasis on platform technologies that either allow for the development of broad-spectrum MCMs, or permit more rapid development of agent-specific countermeasures. Additionally, NIH will focus on MCMs with commercial applicability for routine public health diseases of both domestic and international significance.

NIH and BARDA use Technology Readiness Levels (TRLs),[25] which track product development stages, to coordinate development projects, provide seamless programmatic transition, and ensure continuity of funding for the development of critical MCMs as they mature. NIH will typically carry development efforts through TRL 6 (including clinical Phase I studies), while BARDA picks up development of priority MCMs in TRLs 6-7 (following Phase I).

NIH will also invest in development efforts at early TRL levels to address at-risk population needs and enhance the characteristics of current MCMs that will yield improved impact on end-user needs. Multiple products, some of which have already been placed in the SNS, have successfully transitioned into advanced development through this process. BARDA will continue to support preclinical development (TRL 5) of certain MCMs to address radiological, nuclear, and chemical threats due to the unique features of these threats and the wide array of novel approaches.

Table 2. NIH Near- and Mid-Term Research Priorities

Threats	Research Priorities
Biological (intentional or naturally emerging diseases and pandemic influenza)19	(1.3.4a) Therapeutics, including broad-spectrum antimicrobials, immunomodulators, and host-based therapeutics for bacterial and viral threats
	(1.3.4b) Vaccines with post-exposure prophylactic potential and those that provide enhancements to allow for more effective utilization in public health emergencies
	(1.3.4c) Development of vaccine-related technologies such as adjuvants, temperature stabilization, and alternative delivery devices to enhance the performance, life cycle costs, and utilization/operational capacity for existing biodefense vaccines, with applicability to other infectious diseases or public health situations
	(1.3.4d) Diagnostic platforms and biomarkers
	(1.3.4e) Development and utilization of animal models to support FDA licensure or approval under the Animal Rule,20 as well as to inform utilization policy and optimal treatment regimens (e.g., antibiotic course-duration shortening when combined with vaccination)
Radiological/nuclear	(1.3.4f) Mechanisms of radiation injury at the system, organ, cellular, and molecular levels, with particular focus on the
(intentional or accidental)	hematopoietic, gastrointestinal, immune, pulmonary, renal, and nervous systems, and skin
	(1.3.4g) Approaches to minimize short- and long-term adverse health effects of radiation exposure, including cytokines, growth factors, anti-apoptotics, anti-inflammatory candidates, and antioxidants
	(1.3.4h) Identification and evaluation of biomarkers of radiation injury for use in biodosimetry and bioassay systems for rapid triage, radiation dose estimation, predictive effects on particular organ systems, and extended health risk assessments over time; these will be developed into high-throughput modalities for use in a mass-casualty incident
	(1.3.4i) Identification and development of novel decorporation and blocking agents that prevent the uptake and/or increase the elimination of radionuclides of concern
Chemical (intentional or accidental)	(1.3.4j) Elucidation of mechanisms of chemical injury at the system, organ, cell, and molecular levels, with particular focus on chemicals affecting the nervous system, respiratory tract, skin, eyes and mucous membranes, and cellular respiration
	(1.3.4k) Identification and characterization of approaches to minimize short- and long-term adverse health effects of chemical exposure
	(1.3.4l) MCMs against traditional chemical warfare agents,21 highly toxic industrial chemicals,22 highly toxic agricultural chemicals,23 and poisons

The BARDA CBRN portfolio strategy has evolved over the past eight years to a multi-faceted approach that seeks to:

- Establish public-private and academic-industry partnerships
- Form interagency alliances that enable cost-sharing in the development of key CBRN MCMs
- Develop next-generation MCMs that present improvements over existing ones in regard to effectiveness, ease of administration, cost, and logistics
- Test and evaluate products under development for CBRN indications, those approved for non-CBRN indications that could be repurposed to meet PHEMCE requirements, and multi-purpose product candidates that could meet both PHEMCE requirements and unmet everyday healthcare needs
- Develop innovative technologies to address challenges encountered in CBRN MCM development
- Support host-directed therapeutics[26]
- Establish ready manufacturing capability for pandemic influenza vaccines and other critical MCMs

This emphasis on cross-cutting and platform technologies will greatly enhance the value of U.S. Government (USG) investments by stimulating a more sustainable commercial base for these products, and positioning the PHEMCE to respond more effectively to the unknown threats of the future.

The BARDA influenza portfolio strategy is also focused on developing products with potential for increased effectiveness, greater multi-functionality, and improved operational utility. Examples include advanced development of promising novel and universal vaccine candidates (following proof of concept demonstration in Phase I clinical trials), and development of non-neuraminidase inhibitor therapeutics (including host targets, immune modulators, and drugs used in combination). This approach is also demonstrated in investments toward next- generation ventilators and improvements in respiratory protective devices such that they are reusable, have intuitive fit, and are easy to use by healthcare workers and the public – including pediatric populations – during infectious disease outbreaks. These and other advanced development efforts are described in more detail in Section 3.

(1.3.7) The projected BARDA advanced development and PHEMCE-wide acquisition priorities through FY17, as determined by the PHEMCE prioritization framework, are shown in Table 3. More details on particular programs and timelines are provided in Sections 3 and 4. BARDA is able to both support the advanced development of products, and acquire products for the SNS using the Special Reserve Fund (SRF) authorized under the Project BioShield Act of 2004.[27] Products can be acquired for the SNS by BARDA if/when the product has sufficient safety and efficacy information to permit use under Emergency Use Authorization (EUA) or may reasonably be concluded to qualify for approval, licensing, or clearance within eight years of the decision to procure. MCMs that are already FDA-approved/licensed/ cleared for the desired indication will be available for direct purchase by the CDC.

Table 3. Advanced Development (AD) and Procurement Priorities

Medical Countermeasure Category	*(1.3.7a)* AD Priorities Through FY17[28]	Current HHS Holdings[29]	*(1.3.7b)* Procurements Programmed Through FY13[30]	*(1.3.7c)* Additional Procurements Projected Through FY17[31]
Anthrax Antitoxin	X	X	SRF[32]	TBD[33]
Anthrax Vaccine	X	X	DSNS[34]	DSNS, TBD
Botulism Antitoxin	X	X		
Broad Spectrum Antimicrobials	X	X[35]	DSNS	DSNS, TBD
Cyanide Antidote	X	X		DSNS
Diagnostics – Bioassay	X			
Diagnostics – Biodosimetry	X			TBD
Diagnostics – Biological Agents	X			
Diagnostics – Pandemic Influenza	X			
Diagnostics – Volatile Nerve Agents	X			
Nerve Agent Antidote	X	X	DSNS, SRF	DSNS
Nuclear Agents – Acute Radiation Syndrome (ARS) – Gastrointestinal (GI), Skin, and/or Lung Therapeutics	X			TBD
Nuclear Agents – ARS – Hematopoietic Therapeutics	X	X	SRF	
Nuclear Agents – Thermal Burn Therapeutics	X	X	DSNS	TBD

Medical Countermeasure Category	*(1.3.7a)* AD Priorities Through FY17[28]	Current HHS Holdings[29]	*(1.3.7b)* Procurements Programmed Through FY13[30]	*(1.3.7c)* Additional Procurements Projected Through FY17[31]
Pandemic Influenza Antivirals	X	X	DSNS	DSNS
Pandemic and Pre-Pandemic Influenza Vaccine	X	X		
Patient (Chemical) Decontamination	X			
Radiological Agents – Decorporation/ Blocking Agents	X	X	DSNS	DSNS, TBD
Respiratory Protective Devices	X			DSNS
Smallpox Antivirals	X	X	SRF	
Smallpox Vaccine	X	X	DSNS, SRF	DSNS, TBD
Ventilators	X	X	DSNS	
Viral Hemorrhagic Fever Antivirals	X			
Viral Hemorrhagic Fever Vaccine[36]				

Objective 1.4. Promote effective domestic and international partnerships with developers and manufacturers and support core services. (Leads: ASPR, NIH; Partners: DoD, CDC, FDA, HHS OGA)

Developers and manufacturers of MCMs for the public health emergency threats described in this plan face technical, regulatory, manufacturing, commercialization, and other business challenges that are beyond the resources of many individual private entities. It is important that the USG maintain adequate domestic manufacturing capacity for key medical countermeasures. *(1.4.1)* BARDA will continue to support public-private partnerships with manufacturers to build and/or retrofit medical countermeasure production facilities within the U.S. to increase domestic vaccine and biological therapeutics manufacturing capacity.

To secure a willing and capable partnership with the commercial sector for these unique products, the USG must ensure that these innovators and manufacturers have access to core manufacturing and downstream services to promote the availability of critical MCMs needed to meet civilian requirements. Both NIH and BARDA maintain a wide array of product development and support service contracts that provide infrastructure capabilities for MCM development.[37] *(1.4.2)* The NIH core services[38] cover the spectrum of capabilities that are required for early stages of product development, and include animal model development support, research facilities, manufacturing support, and advice on working with other federal agencies, such as BARDA, DoD, and FDA. In particular, NIH, in conjunction with BARDA, CDC, and DoD partners, works closely with the FDA to pursue development of relevant animal efficacy models in order to facilitate potential Animal Rule approval pathways.

BARDA is now positioned to provide highly significant core-services support to assist MCM developers in various aspects of product testing, development, validation, and production. BARDA recently established the Centers for Innovation in Advanced Development and Manufacturing (CIADMs).[39] *(1.4.3)* BARDA has also established a Nonclinical Product Development Network to provide core services (e.g., product testing, animal model qualification, assay development, and reagent qualification) to product developers to ensure that scientific and regulatory requirements for approval and utilization of MCMs can be met. In addition, BARDA is establishing a domestic Fill-Finish Manufacturing Network to supplement manufacturing of pandemic influenza vaccine and other sterile injectable products needed in an emergency or during shortages. *(1.4.4)* Lastly, BARDA plans to establish a Clinical Research Organization (CRO) Network by late 2014 to allow BARDA to conduct clinical trials with investigational MCMs. The CRO Network will consist of several CROs that are capable of conducting Phase I-IV clinical trials and of expediting clinical trials in the event of a public health emergency.

(1.4.5) PHEMCE partners will also enter into strategic bilateral and multilateral engagements with international partners to identify joint opportunities for product development, including efforts to support the establishment of sustainable international pandemic influenza vaccine production capacity. *(1.4.6)* To that end, BARDA, with the support of OGA, will maintain its financial and technical support of the World Health Organization (WHO) Global Action Plan, working in concert with the Developing Countries Vaccine Manufacturers Network and other partners to expand influenza vaccine manufacturing capacity in developing countries.

GOAL 2. Establish and communicate clear regulatory pathways to facilitate medical countermeasure development and use.

Objective 2.1. Identify scientific and regulatory issues that challenge medical countermeasure development or use during public health emergencies and coordinate activities among PHEMCE partners to address those challenges. (Lead: FDA; Partners: PHEMCE agencies)

(2.1.1) The FDA, through its Medical Countermeasures Initiative (MCMi),[40] will engage with PHEMCE partners in identifying and resolving the regulatory and scientific challenges that impede MCM development and use, based on near-, mid-, and long-term PHEMCE priorities and requirements. The MCMi addresses key challenges in three areas: (1) enhancing FDA's product review and approval processes for the highest-priority MCMs and related technologies; (2) advancing regulatory science to support MCM development and regulatory review; and (3) modernizing the legal, regulatory, and policy framework to facilitate MCM development and availability.[41]

(2.1.2) To enhance the MCM review and approval processes, FDA will establish multidisciplinary Public Health and Security Action Teams (Action Teams) to identify and help resolve regulatory and scientific challenges for high-priority MCMs and related technologies.[42] Since 2011, FDA has established five Action Teams. The work of the Surveillance Action Team, co-led by CDC, is discussed under Objective 3.4. The other Action Teams include:

- *(2.1.2a) Multiplex In Vitro Diagnostic Action Team:* This Action Team is facilitating efforts to establish standards for evaluating multiplex *in vitro* diagnostic tests. In 2011, FDA published a concept paper on novel regulatory approaches for multiplex diagnostic tests and convened a workshop on advancing regulatory science for highly multiplexed microbiology/MCM devices. *(2.1.2a1) (2.1.2a1)* These efforts helped clarify the regulatory pathway for developing multiplex diagnostic devices, and FDA will use this information to provide regulatory support in the near term on the topic. FDA will also collaborate with the Defense Threat Reduction Agency, the National Library of Medicine, and the National Institute of Standards and Technology to establish a publicly availablereference database that will be critical to developers seeking to validate their candidate multiplex *in vitro* diagnostic tests.
- *(2.1.2b) Acute Radiation Syndrome (ARS)/Biodosimetry Action Team:* This Action Team will facilitate the development and regulatory review

of MCMs for ARS indications. For example, to date this Action Team has facilitated the completion of a pre-EUA[43] package for an ARS product held in the SNS. *(2.1.2b1)* This Action Team will continue to clarify the regulatory pathway for candidate ARS products in the BARDA pipeline. *(2.1.2b2)* In addition, this Action Team will work to facilitate the development and regulatory review of biodosimetry devices and will continue to provide regulatory support on establishing the performance of radiation biodosimetry devices.

- *(2.1.2c) Warfighter-Trauma Action Team*: This Action Team is facilitating the development and evaluation of MCMs and related technologies to support the warfighter and trauma victims. This Action Team will collaborate with DoD to identify programs, products, and technologies of high-priority for the DoD, and will provide assistance on selected regulatory and policy issues, including pre-EUA package development, to facilitate their continued development or availability.
- *(2.1.2d) Pediatrics and Maternal Action Team:* This Action Team will work to ensure that the MCM needs of at-risk populations, and specifically pediatric and maternal populations, can be met during public health emergencies. For example, this Action Team is discussing potential data gaps with CDC that could inhibit the effective use of stockpiled MCMs in children and other at-risk populations. *(2.1.2d1)* FDA will work with PHEMCE partners to fill those data gaps.

FDA will sustain these Action Teams as necessary through FY17 and will establish new Action Teams as needed based on evolving PHEMCE priorities.

FDA will also build the science base necessary to support MCM development and regulatory assessment through the Medical Countermeasure Regulatory Science Program.[44] The MCM Regulatory Science Program includes both an internal FDA component and an external, collaborative component that focuses on partnerships with USG agencies, academia, non-governmental organizations (NGOs), and industry. To date, more than 90 unique regulatory research proposals spanning FDA's three product review centers – the Centers for Biologics Evaluation and Research (CBER), Drug Evaluation and Research (CDER), and Devices and Radiological Health (CDRH) – have been funded.[45] Additionally, external partnerships to facilitate the development of MCMs are being established through the FDA Advancing Regulatory Science and Innovation Broad Agency Announcement. *(2.1.3)* In the near term, FDA will work closely with PHEMCE partners to identify MCM regulatory science needs. *(2.1.4)* FDA will focus on critical gaps and emerging technologies, including developing and qualifying tools to assess efficacy, such as animal and biomimetic models; developing methods to assess product quality and assays to support the deployment of MCMs; developing and assessing advanced diagnostic tests; and developing novel manufacturing platforms. *(2.1.5)* FDA will also establish a partners program in the near term to link FDA scientists with extramural partners to pursue cutting-edge regulatory science projects.

(2.1.6) Other PHEMCE partners also fund regulatory science projects and work closely to identify and fill priority data gaps related to stockpiled MCMs and other needs, fostering rapid response and maximizing preparedness. *(2.1.7)* PHEMCE partners will work with the FDA's Drug Development Tool (DDT) Qualification Program[46] to develop tools – such as animal models and biomarkers – facilitating MCM development and identifying and filling priority data gaps.

(2.1.8) FDA has also established a policy team that works closely with the Action Teams to ensure that FDA laws, regulations, and policies adequately support MCM development, distribution, administration, and use. Where changes are needed to better protect public health, FDA works with appropriate partners to develop and propose new approaches.[47] FDA analyzed the existing statutory framework for making MCMs available in emergency circumstances, and based on this analysis, developed proposals for the Pandemic and All Hazards Preparedness Reauthorization Act (PAHPRA). If enacted, the changes would enhance clarity and flexibility for use of the EUA authority, as well as for certain uses of approved, licensed, or cleared MCMs. *(2.1.9)* Should PAHPRA become law, FDA will provide guidance to stakeholders and implement FDA-related statutory changes, such as by updating the current EUA Guidance, to optimize our country's ability to efficiently and effectively prepare for and respond to public health emergencies. *(2.1.10)* In addition, FDA will provide policy assistance for relevant partners as necessary on issues including first responders' ready access to and use of MCMs; MCM development challenges that are unique to the warfighter; expiration dating as it pertains uniquely to stockpiled MCMs; data collection during a public health emergency; guidance development (e.g., for multiplex *in vitro* diagnostics and implementation of the Animal Rule); and import and export during emergency responses.

Objective 2.2. Assist medical countermeasure developers in working interactively with FDA during product development and regulatory review. (Lead: FDA; Partners: NIH, ASPR)

The PHEMCE is committed to assisting MCM developers in navigating the USG MCM regulatory assessment and review processes. *(2.2.1)* FDA will assist in the clarification of regulatory pathways and reduction of regulatory barriers using the following methods:

- Formal and informal meetings with product sponsors or applicants seeking technical assistance related to the development, regulatory assessment of MCMs, and manufacturing
- Enhanced inspection, including pre-approval, and compliance activities to support early identification of problems that might impede MCM development
- Issuance of guidance documents and rules and regulations based on the laws that FDA enforces to help foster MCM development and availability
- Stakeholder engagements, including meetings, conferences, and workshops, to educate the public on both FDA regulatory processes and its current thinking on regulatory issues, and to garner input from interested parties on regulatory issues
- Public Advisory Committee meetings to obtain independent expert advice on scientific, technical, and policy matters on specific topics

NIH and BARDA will provide product development core services to developers and manufacturers, as described in Objective 1.4, to assist in the regulatory process. *(2.2.2)* BARDA and NIH will develop and qualify animal models through the new Animal Model Development Program, and perform efficacy evaluations in compliance with Good Laboratory Practice (GLP) requirements and testing of CBRN countermeasures in qualified animal models. *(2.2.3)* BARDA subject matter experts will assist private-sector partners in the development of regulatory strategies, including the design and execution of pivotal animal studies and clinical studies, preparation of regulatory documentation, and strategic communication on regulatory issues.

GOAL 3. Develop logistics and operational plans for optimized use of medical countermeasures at all levels of response.

Objective 3.1 Promote innovative approaches to inventory management to enable a sustainable preparedness infrastructure. (Lead: CDC; Partners: ASPR, DHS)

The PHEMCE will focus on issues of long-term sustainability and enhanced flexibility to ensure cost-effectiveness of federal MCM stockpiles while maintaining readiness. This will be accomplished through: (1) optimizing the SNS formulary; (2) ensuring cost-effective formulary management; and (3) examining novel inventory management mechanisms that ensure timely access to needed medical products.

Optimization of the SNS Formulary

(3.1.1) The PHEMCE SNS Annual Review represents a continuous process for optimizing the contents of the SNS. The Review, required by both statute[48] and Executive Order,[49] comprehensively examines the SNS formulary each year, including non-pharmaceutical countermeasures and ancillary supplies; identifies and prioritizes formulary gaps; and recommends additions or modifications to the contents of the SNS, in alignment with the PHEMCE prioritization framework. (3.1.2) Over the near term, the PHEMCE will develop a risk-based analysis of investment needs by leveraging perspectives from the intelligence community and DHS risk assessment processes. This two-year project will inform the optimization of SNS contents by demonstrating how particular formulary options may decrease the risk against CBRN threats. (3.1.3) The PHEMCE is also actively exploring alternatives to central stockpiling as appropriate, such as "just-in-time" manufacturing and/or procurement, support for surge manufacturing capabilities, stockpiling of bulk product, and alternative stockpiling options such as rotated inventory, home or business caching, and/or other vendor- or user-managed inventory approaches.

Cost-Effective Management of SNS Assets

(3.1.4) CDC will effectively and efficiently maintain, replace, and manage assets in the SNS across their life-cycles to ensure they can be accessed and provided when and where needed, within operational and logistical constraints.

To accomplish these functions, the CDC will utilize a robust inventory management system, including state-of-the-art monitoring systems, Quality Control Unit evaluation of storage facilities, and comprehensive annual inventories and inventory tracking mechanisms. MCMs requiring rapid administration for clinically effective use may be held in forward-placed or prepackaged storage for ready access.[50]

(3.1.5) CDC will also continue to participate in the FDA/DoD Shelf Life Extension Program (SLEP)[51] to extend the viability of appropriate stockpiled products when it is cost- effective, to improve efficiency and to maximize existing investments.

(3.1.6) Finally, over the near and mid terms, CDC will examine ways to reduce the time required to deploy assets at the federal level, and better understand the costs at the federal and SLTT levels.

Long-Term Sustainability

(3.1.7) While many of the previously mentioned actions will support long-term sustainability of the SNS, ASPR and CDC have also charged the National Biodefense Science Board (NBSB)[52] and the Board of Scientific Counselors (BSC) of the CDC Office of Public Health Preparedness and Response (PHPR)[53] to (1) identify the anticipated responsibilities of the SNS in the year 2020; (2) recommend approaches for meeting those responsibilities as efficiently as possible; and (3) propose metrics for reporting program capability and informing improvement. The results of these deliberations are anticipated by the end of FY13, and will be incorporated into ongoing SNS budgeting and planning once available.

Objective 3.2 Develop and communicate medical countermeasure utilization policy, guidance and response strategies, including FDA regulatory frameworks, that are responsive to end-user needs and that are integrated with state, local, tribal, territorial (SLTT) and private sector response plans, and when possible international partners, and that ensure timely, safe, and effective medical countermeasure distribution and utilization. (Leads: ASPR, CDC; Partners: PHEMCE agencies)

Linking Bench to Community (Leads: ASPR, NIH)

End-user needs are key drivers in MCM development. For example, NIH early research into vaccine adjuvants is aimed not only at increasing vaccine efficacy, but also at developing a faster onset of protection with fewer vaccine doses, resulting in decreased stockpiling costs and improved response logistics. Similarly, NIH research into temperature stabilization for critical MCMs may decrease or eliminate the need for cold chain storage, decreasing stockpiling costs and widening distribution options in an emergency.

(3.2.1) In the advanced development of priority MCMs, BARDA will work with developers to ensure that MCM development plans take into account the most up-to-date utilization policies, response strategies, evolving regulatory guidance for use, and other relevant factors. Strengthening this feedback loop between the end-users and the developers of MCMs will result in products that can be most effectively used in public health emergencies.

Developing Additional Federal Operational and Response Plans (Leads: ASPR, CDC; Partners: PHEMCE Agencies)

(3.2.2) Over the next five years, the PHEMCE, through the leadership of the CDC and ASPR, and as supported by other USG partners and external experts,[54] will leverage the lessons learned at all levels from previous incident responses to develop and share MCM response strategies, utilization guidances, CONOPs, and clinical practice guidelines with end-users as appropriate. (3.2.3) ASPR will collaborate with PHEMCE partners to ensure MCM plans and clinical guidelines are appropriately captured in the federal all-hazards emergency response planning process and also contribute to regional operational planning. Through ongoing collaborative efforts with PHEMCE partners and external stakeholders, the FDA will work to modernize the legal, regulatory, and policy frameworks to facilitate the development and availability of MCMs; enhance pre-event planning; and foster rapid MCM deployment and use in public health emergencies. (3.2.4) CDC will collaborate with DHS, FDA, and BARDA to establish a process to validate laboratory methods and enhance national capacity to rapidly test clinical specimens and determine who has been exposed to biological agents. These efforts will enable the public health community to respond effectively and appropriately to provide timely post-exposure prophylaxis (PEP) and general public health interventions. (3.2.5) CDC, DHS, and DoD will develop rapid antimicrobial resistance testing to quickly identify agents that may be resistant to first-line MCMs in the SNS, allowing real-time course corrections in response strategies and MCM utilization plans.

(3.2.6) More specifically, over the course of this Implementation Plan, the PHEMCE will develop the following deliverables to facilitate national public health emergency response for high-priority threats:

- *(3.2.6a)* National smallpox vaccine and anthrax response strategies, including prioritization schemes in the case of limited resources (FY13)
- *(3.2.6b)* Clinical practice guidelines for MCMs to address smallpox, anthrax, melioidosis, glanders, ARS-associated neutropenia,[55] and chemical agents (near-, mid-, and longterm completion)
- *(3.2.6c)* Assessment of state and local capacity to utilize cytokines for ARS-associated neutropenia following use of an improvised nuclear device (FY13)
- *(3.2.6d)* Decision-making and planning guidance for dispensing models to meet the diverse needs of communities (near-term completion)
- *(3.2.6e)* End-user handbook(s) for various stakeholders that will include: response strategies, MCM CONOPs, utilization guidances, and clinical practice guidelines to ensure that the information in MCM response integration and utilization plans will be readily accessible in an emergency (mid- to long-term completion)
- *(3.2.6f)* Planning guidance for patient decontamination in a mass exposure chemical incident (FY13)

Adding to Key Federal Policy and Response Capabilities (Lead: ASPR)

ASPR is also leading several initiatives to ensure preparedness in key functional areas critical for an effective national response:

- *(3.2.7) Emergency Policy Coordination:* ASPR has established the Disaster Leadership Group (DLG) as the mechanism to ensure a coordinated, Department-wide, strategic approach to HHS emergency response and recovery efforts among the executive leadership of the Department. As the Secretary's principal advisor on all matters related to public health and medical emergency preparedness and response, the ASPR will chair and convene the DLG in a public health emergency to discuss, coordinate, and promote approaches to address the policy, budget, legislative, and external communication strategies and needs associated with the response. The DLG will identify and resolve policy issues and potential barriers, including those related to MCM production, distribution, dispensing/administration, and use, which may directly impact effective response operations during specific emergency events.

- *(3.2.8) Fiscal and Administrative Preparedness:* Recent public health emergencies such as 2009 H1N1 pandemic influenza and the 2010 Gulf oil spill highlighted the need for a much more responsive fiscal and administrative framework to most effectively utilize resources during an emergency. *(3.2.8a)* In support of the MCM-related aspects of this larger effort, ASPR will ensure that the fiscal and administrative practices to rapidly produce and effectively distribute MCMs are incorporated into pre-event planning activities. *(3.2.8b)* In the near term, the PHEMCE, through collaboration with finance, budget, and contract management partners, will identify strategies to accelerate the MCM-related administrative decision-making processes. This will be accomplished by informing the budget estimation process for MCM needs; ensuring end-to-end communication regarding accessing financial resources; engaging in post-event accountability evaluations related to MCM budget and financial processes; and contributing to the development of mechanisms to better understand and articulate funding utilization.
- *(3.2.9) Science Preparedness:* ASPR will lead an initiative to coordinate science preparedness and response efforts across the diverse span of interagency emergency preparedness efforts, including those related to MCMs. Research before, during, and after an emergency is critical to our future capacity to better prevent injury, illness, disability, and death, while supporting recovery. This effort can also ensure that the appropriate subject matter experts from government, academic institutions, non- governmental organizations, and the private sector can be leveraged to assist in response to a public health emergency. Over the next five years, ASPR will focus on areas such as clinical protocols and datasets, specimens, workforce, policies, rapid funding mechanisms for research, and surveys.

Support for SLTT Response Efforts (Leads: CDC, ASPR; Partner: FDA)

The PHEMCE will work with all stakeholders, including SLTT authorities, community groups, and professional societies, to develop and implement mechanisms to achieve timely access to MCMs for those who need them. *(3.2.10)* Throughout the next five years, the CDC, in collaboration with ASPR, will provide guidance to SLTT partners on receiving and effectively utilizing (i.e., deploying, distributing, and dispensing) MCMs provided by the SNS. *(3.2.11)* ASPR will collaborate broadly with PHEMCE and non-federal partners, to include regional healthcare coalitions and state authorities, to develop resilient systems of care that will be able to optimally respond to and recover from public health emergencies. Such efforts will include direct funding support, as well as initiatives aimed at building MCM delivery and utilization capabilities at the regional level, including the National Postal Model (NPM)[56] and Hospital Preparedness Program (HPP).[57]

International Efforts (Lead: ASPR; Partners: FDA, CDC, HHS OGA, USDA)

While the PHEMCE focus is predominantly on meeting U.S. domestic MCM needs, utilization policies, clinical guidances, and response strategies should be integrated with those of our international partners where appropriate. Building on the lessons learned during the 2009 H1N1 influenza pandemic and the nuclear power plant incident in Fukushima in 2011, the PHEMCE will identify and address barriers to building a sustainable global infrastructure for MCMs. *(3.2.12)* Domestically, and in collaboration with all USG stakeholders, ASPR will develop and implement a strategic policy framework over the next two years to respond to international requests for MCMs and to accept assistance from foreign countries. *(3.2.13)* In parallel, ASPR and other relevant HHS agencies will continue to engage international partners to identify joint opportunities for product development, and will collaborate with WHO and the Global Health Security Initiative (GHSI) partners[58] to overcome barriers and develop protocols to facilitate the international deployment and distribution of MCMs during public health emergencies. *(3.2.14)* Regionally, ASPR will work with Canada and Mexico over the next three years to overcome barriers to providing mutual assistance and harmonize utilization policies for MCMs during international public health emergencies under the framework of the U.S.-Canada Beyond the Border Initiative,[59] and as called for in the North American Plan for Animal and Pandemic Influenza.[60]

Objective 3.3. Develop and provide medical countermeasure communications, training, and education information to inform all stakeholders. (Leads: CDC, ASPR; Partners: FDA, USDA)

As stated in the NHSS,[61] the PHEMCE will ensure effective communications with both responders and the public through the timely release of credible, understandable, and actionable information both prior to and during public health emergencies.

(3.3.1) Over the next three years, the PHEMCE will develop a comprehensive medical countermeasure messaging program and multi-year implementation plan. This program will ensure that messaging protocols and data sources across the various response organizations are clearly defined. The PHEMCE will work with partners to expand message content to stakeholders and make national health security messages (covering such topics as preparedness, response, and recovery) available in multiple formats and languages. As part of this process, the PHEMCE will establish and implement a press release development policy whereby a standard operating procedure and centralized talking points will be used to ensure consistent messaging by both deployed teams and PHEMCE leadership during a response.

(3.3.2) The CDC, in coordination with FDA and ASPR, will test the effectiveness of MCM-related public health communication materials through focus groups and other methods. *(3.3.3)* ASPR will provide training for the National Disaster Medical System (NDMS) workforce on the use of MCMs against all hazards, including making available just-in-time advanced training for MCMs targeting particular threat agents.

(3.3.4) In addition, ASPR will develop and implement a plan to disseminate best practices for establishing and maintaining regional coordination for public health emergencies. Specifically, the PHEMCE will promote partnerships over the next two years among emergency management, healthcare, behavioral healthcare, and human services stakeholders by providing technical assistance and education to SLTT and non-governmental partners in a sustainable, scheduled forum.

Objective 3.4. Develop and implement strategies to assess, evaluate, and monitor medical countermeasure safety, performance, and patient compliance during and after a public health emergency response. (Leads: FDA, CDC, ASPR)

(3.4.1) FDA and CDC co-lead the Surveillance Action Team charged with identifying the regulatory science research required of realǦtime tracking and evaluation of MCMs during public health emergencies. The Action Team will develop, in the near term, a comprehensive Action Plan to identify and facilitate the development of systems that can be used to monitor MCM safety and clinical benefit during an event. *(3.4.2)* Other PHEMCE agencies, including BARDA, will be joining FDA and CDC in moving forward in the mid-term to implement these systems, as called for in the Action Plan.

GOAL 4. Address medical countermeasure gaps for all sectors of the American civilian population.

The PHEMCE considers the needs of at-risk populations throughout all of the activities described in Goals 1-3 above. This sub-section describes activities specifically directed at addressing at-risk population needs.

Objective 4.1. Develop medical consequence and public health response assessments and requirements setting for at-risk individuals. (Lead: ASPR; Partners: PHEMCE agencies)

(4.1.1) PHEMCE requirement-setting, as detailed in Objective 1.2 above, will assess at-risk population needs at every stage of the process. Additionally, BARDA has collated the existing, albeit limited, clinical and scientific literature on agent susceptibility and MCM utility in these populations. At-risk populations such as children, pregnant women, elderly adults, and those with underlying medical conditions potentially have differences in susceptibility to CBRN agents, and/or altered disease severity following exposure. In many cases, the first-line treatments for CBRN agents have not been tested, or are not recommended for use, in at-risk populations. (4.1.2) Important gaps in the scientific knowledge of these at-risk group differences exist, and the PHEMCE will support research efforts to close these gaps, in alignment with the prioritization criteria detailed previously, and as ethically feasible.[62] This data collection will inform utilization of current MCMs and the desired characteristics of future products.

(4.1.3) As data become available, BARDA will update its public health and medical consequence models to estimate pediatric and other at-risk population MCM needs, including consideration of MCM contraindications or the impact of not authorizing their use in these populations during an emergency response.

(4.1.4) The PHEMCE has established a Pediatric and Obstetric Integrated Program Team (PedsOB IPT). The PedsOB IPT will provide subject matter expertise for developing MCM requirements and strategies, and for promotion of the availability of pediatric[63] and obstetric MCMs in public health emergencies. Notably, formulations suitable for pediatric and obstetric populations may also benefit other at-risk groups. For example, in parallel with its evaluation of the minimum practical age for using crushed tablets instead of more expensive antibiotic suspensions in pediatric populations, the PedsOB IPT also considered use of these suspension formulations for geriatric populations and people who have difficulty swallowing.

Objective 4.2. Support medical countermeasure advanced development and procurement for at-risk individuals. (Leads: ASPR, NIH, FDA; Partner: CDC)

HHS currently holds a large amount of MCMs that can potentially be used in particular at-risk populations, albeit often only under regulatory mechanisms such as Investigational New Drug (IND) protocols or EUAs. Box 1 lists the currently stockpiled MCMs that can potentially be used in pediatric populations, along with the threats those countermeasures address.

Box 1. Stockpiled Medical Countermeasures Potentially Available for Use in Pediatric Populations

- Oral Solid and Liquid Antimicrobials – *Anthrax, Plague, Tularemia, Typhus*
- IV Antimicrobials – *Anthrax, Plague, Tularemia, Pandemic Influenza", Radiological and Nuclear Threats", Typhus*
- Vaccines – *Anthrax, Smallpox, Pandemic Influenza*
- Antitoxins or Immunoglobulins – *Anthrax, Botulism, Smallpox*
- Oral and IV Chelators – *Radiological Threats*
- Hematopoietic Agents – *Radiological and Nuclear Threats*
- Thermal Burn Supplies – *Radiological and NuclearThreats*

- Nerve Agent and Cyanide Antidotes – *Chemical Threats*
- Oral Solid Antivirals – *Smallpox, Pandemic Influenza*
- Inhaled and Oral Liquid Antivirals – *Pandemic Influenza*
- IV Antivirals – *Smallpox, Radiological and Nuclear Threats*[^], *Pandemic Influenza*
- Ventilators – *All Hazards*

^for secondary infections

The PHEMCE will support MCM development and FDA approval/licensure/clearance to address the needs of at-risk populations, including expansion of label indications and/or development of new formulations as needed. Specifically, the PHEMCE will implement the following initiatives:

- *(4.2.1)* BARDA will support studies to develop pediatric and geriatric indications and formulations as needed in all MCM late-stage development and procurement contracts. BARDA contracts for product development also include considerations of safety in pregnant women and immunocompromised individuals. (ongoing)
- *(4.2.2)* In the area of off-patent, approved drugs being pursued for additional CBRN indications, NIH and FDA have specifically identified products for which pediatric safety databases exist, and will focus efforts to assess existing data necessary to demonstrate efficacy for pediatric populations using those data without the need for additional studies in these populations. (near-term)
- *(4.2.3)* At-risk population needs are explicitly taken into account through the SNS Annual Review. Appropriate products or formulations for these groups, and/or suitable operational alternatives, will be advanced when available and as resources allow. (ongoing)
- *(4.2.4)* FDA will sponsor workshops on the ethical and regulatory challenges in the development of pediatric MCMs, and the scientific issues related to selecting animal models for use in evaluating products that may be used during pregnancy. (ongoing)
- *(4.2.5)* BARDA, working with CDC, will support efforts to achieve FDA licensure (in healthy populations) for a smallpox vaccine that is ultimately intended for use in immunocompromised individuals in an emergency. (ongoing)

Objective 4.3. Develop and implement strategies, policies, and guidance to support the appropriate use of medical countermeasures in all civilian populations during an emergency. (Leads: ASPR, CDC; Partner: FDA)

To support the use of stockpiled MCMs in at-risk populations, in the near- and mid-terms, the PHEMCE will pursue policies and programs related to regulatory challenges associated with products intended for at-risk populations, including filling priority data gaps associated with developing pre-EUA packages to support the use of stockpiled MCMs in these populations.

(4.3.1) In the near to mid terms, The PHEMCE will provide clinicians with dosing and use guidance for using stockpiled MCMs in pediatric populations (such as amoxicillin and other antimicrobial agents, anthrax antitoxin, anthrax vaccine, and Prussian blue in infants less than two years of age), with the caveat that this guidance could only be used in an emergency (e.g., under an EUA).

(4.3.2) In the near term, the PHEMCE will establish a means to ensure that public health and medical information distributed during public health emergencies is delivered in a manner that takes into account the range of communication and other functional needs of the intended recipients, including at-risk individuals. The information will be disseminated to end-users before, during, and following public health emergencies in as timely a manner as practicable, and updated as appropriate. This information will incorporate best practices for outreach to, and care of, at-risk individuals. CDC guidance provided to federal and SLTT partners on MCM distribution and dispensing/administration, as described under Objective 3.2, will likewise include consideration of at-risk population needs. (4.3.3) The PHEMCE will leverage its established relationships with the American Academy of Pediatrics and other clinical organizations serving the needs of at-risk populations to help inform MCM strategies and policies related to these groups.

(4.3.4) ASPR and the Administration for Children and Families (ACF) established the Children's HHS Interagency Leadership on Disasters (CHILD) Working Group in 2010 to identify and comprehensively integrate departmental activities related to the needs of children across all HHS inter- and intra-governmental disaster planning initiatives and operations. The CHILD Working Group, which includes representatives from ASPR, CDC,

FDA, and NIH, developed six recommendations specific to pediatric MCM needs in its 2011 report, several of which have already been implemented.[64]

ASPR will also focus resources toward anticipating and addressing the needs of at-risk populations during a disaster as follows:

- *(4.3.5)* ASPR's NDMS has a pediatrician serving as its director. During an emergency, NDMS will assist/supplement state and local MCM distribution and dispensing efforts as needed, including those aimed at pediatric and other at-risk populations.
- *(4.3.6)* ASPR's Emergency Care Coordination Center (ECCC) is now led by a former member of the National Commission on Children and Disasters.[65] Over the mid term, the ECCC will examine the systemic issues that could affect MCM dispensing to at-risk populations.
- *(4.3.7)* ASPR, through its engagement and support of the Federal Education and Training Interagency Group and the National Center for Disaster Medicine and Public Health, will support the development of pediatric-specific training curriculum guidance for managing children's needs in times of disasters. (ongoing)
- *(4.3.8)* The ASPR Playbooks for each National Planning Scenario, which outline key options and actions to aid the HHS Secretary and the ASPR in making necessary decisions in an emergency, will integrate operational considerations, resources, and action items targeting the needs of pediatric and other at-risk populations. (near-term)

SECTION 2: INTERAGENCY PARTNER ROLES AND COLLABORATIONS IN SUPPORTING STRATEGIC GOALS AND OBJECTIVES

As stated in the *2012 PHEMCE Strategy*, accomplishing the established goals and objectives will require the coordination of MCM-related activities across multiple Federal departments. Key PHEMCE interagency partners to HHS in this endeavor include DHS, DoD, VA, and USDA. The critical roles these agencies play, and will continue to exercise, in support of these goals and objectives are detailed below.

Department of Homeland Security

DHS leads the Federal response to incidents involving interagency and multi-jurisdictional response. DHS has the responsibility for developing and conducting threat and risk assessment processes that integrate the findings of the intelligence and law enforcement communities with input from the scientific, medical, and public health communities to inform investment priorities for current and anticipated threats. DHS identifies high-risk threats that hold potential for catastrophic consequences to civilian populations and warrant development of targeted countermeasures. *(I.1)* Pursuant to the Project BioShield Act of 2004, DHS will continue to use this capability to make determinations about which CBRN agents pose a material threat sufficient to affect U.S. national security. *(I.2)* DHS will further advance this capability to provide strategic, integrated all-CBRN risk assessments to facilitate prioritization of MCM development across the CBRN threat spectrum. The Secretaries of DHS and HHS must jointly recommend the use of the SRF created under Project BioShield to the Director of the Office of Management and Budget, acting on behalf of the President, prior to its use.

Department of Defense

The Secretary of Defense has primary responsibility for the research, development, acquisition, and deployment of MCMs for the Armed Forces. DoD will continue to direct strategic planning for and oversight of programs to support MCM development and acquisition for armed forces personnel. *(I.3)* Through their work in the PHEMCE, DoD and HHS will coordinate their efforts to promote synergy, minimize redundancy, and, to the extent feasible, harmonize requirements for MCM development. DoD will continue to draw upon its longstanding investment and experience in CBRN MCM research, development, acquisition, and deployment to ensure protection of the Armed Forces, and also to accelerate and improve the overall national effort, consistent with DoD authorities and responsibilities. *(I.4)* DoD will continue to place a special focus on MCM development for CBRN threats due to the unique facilities, testing capabilities, and trained and experienced personnel available at DoD for this purpose. *(I.5)* HHS and DoD will continue to coordinate on the research, development, and procurement of safe and effective MCMs of mutual interest. For example, the DoD and HHS advanced research and development programs for CBRN MCMs are closely coordinated through the PHEMCE Integrated Portfolio for CBRN MCMs, a group that is co-led by both departments and comprises program representatives from the various organizations responsible for the CBRN MCM programs within each department. DoD and HHS further cooperate on the procurement of specific MCMs through interdepartmental agreements and fund transfers.

Department of Veterans Affairs

VA serves a critical role in its mission of providing health care to the Veteran population, as well as providing support to DoD and the nation in times of emergencies impacting public health. *(I.6)* VA coordinates with DHS and HHS to promote synergy, minimize redundancy, and use common requirements for MCMs to ensure the VA can continue to fulfill its mission. *(I.7)* The VA also provides contracting services for the SNS.

Department of Agriculture

USDA leads federal government efforts to protect against any agent that poses a threat to plant or animal health.[66] These efforts protect public health as it relates to the adulteration of food and other products regulated by the Secretary of Agriculture. These efforts also address the environment as it relates to agriculture facilities, farmland, and air and water within the immediate vicinity of an agricultural disease or outbreak. More broadly, USDA leads in the research, development, and licensure of products, practices, technologies, or other agricultural countermeasures (i.e., those not used solely in response to a human medical incident or in a non- agriculture-related public health emergency) necessary to enhance or maintain the agricultural biosecurity of the U.S. In particular, USDA has research activities specifically focused on veterinary countermeasures, and maintains veterinary countermeasure stockpiles analogous to the SNS. *(I.8)* Also, USDA coordinates with HHS, through the FDA Commissioner and the CDC Director, on the surveillance of zoonotic diseases. USDA has established a One Health initiative[67] that provides a focal point for the Department to comprehensively consider and address zoonotic threats.

SECTION 3: THREAT-BASED APPROACHES

The PHEMCE recognizes the need to address the high-priority threats identified in the Strategy. While the PHEMCE is evolving toward capability-based approaches, it will maintain key threat-based approaches needed to address these threats to national health security. This section describes in detail the activities and programs that were prioritized based on the PHEMCE prioritization framework to support the threat-based approaches described in the body of this document.

ANTHRAX

The HHS PHEMCE anthrax programmatic priorities include:

- Increasing the currently licensed vaccine's utility for PEP
- Streamlining the currently licensed vaccine's administration requirements
- Reducing vaccine lifecycle costs
- Developing next-generation anthrax vaccine candidates
- Providing and maintaining enough vaccine regimens for the SNS to meet the established PHEMCE goal
- Enhancing the utility of anthrax vaccines by lowering cost per dose
- Encouraging competition among product sponsors
- Building in redundancy to mitigate risk
- Investing in novel expression and manufacturing platform technologies that are readily transferrable before or after a public health emergency to increase production capacity for anthrax vaccine

Near-term (FY12-14)

Anthrax Clinical Guidance and Communication Materials

The Anthrax Management Team (AMT) was established in 2010 to coordinate, consolidate and integrate all anthrax-related activities at the CDC. When these activities involve MCMs, the activities of this team will be guided by the PHEMCE prioritization framework described in this Plan. *(T.A.1)* The AMT will complete several stakeholder engagements and subject matter expert meetings to inform an updated anthrax clinical guidance for all populations. *(T.A.2)* This will be followed in the mid term by the publication of an updated anthrax clinical guidance. *(T.A.3)* CDC will also develop risk-communication materials for an anthrax incident.

Anthrax Vaccine

(T.A.4) NIH is focusing on improving the currently licensed anthrax vaccine through the development and testing of adjuvants that could enhance performance and reduce the doses necessary to achieve full immunity in a pre-exposure setting. Human clinical testing is underway, with advanced development anticipated by FY14. *(T.A.5)* BARDA will support advanced development to expand the vaccine's indications to include PEP, and work to extend product expiry. *(T.A.6)* NIH, CDC and FDA, working with the vaccine manufacturer, are supporting research into dose-sparing strategies for PEP vaccine use, with completion anticipated in FY13. *(T.A.7)* BARDA will also support investigation of the vaccine's impact on the pharmacokinetics of those antimicrobials that would be used in combination with it for PEP, while the vaccine manufacturer is researching these antimicrobials' impact on vaccine immunogenicity under PEP conditions. *(T.A.8)* Furthermore, BARDA will continue development of existing recombinant anthrax protective antigen (rPA) vaccine candidates in its pipeline. *(T.A.9)* In the meantime, CDC, working with FDA, will complete the anthrax vaccine prioritization guidance.

Anthrax Antitoxin

(T.A.10) BARDA will support the pursuit of FDA approval for the most advanced-stage anthrax antitoxins, including late-stage development and deliveries to the SNS. (T.A.11) BARDA will also support late-stage development of an alternative antitoxin. (T.A.12) BARDA will develop investigational plans to collect clinical data in at-risk populations during mass-casualty events. (T.A.13) In addition, BARDA, in coordination with CDC, will initiate antitoxin-related outreach, communication, and education programs with Regional Emergency Coordinators (RECs)[68] and ASPR recovery planners.

Anthrax Antimicrobials and Diagnostics

(T.A.14) Animal model testing to support approval for use against inhalational anthrax of antimicrobials currently approved for other indications is in progress at NIH, with FDA review anticipated in FY13. Additional antimicrobial development efforts are also underway at NIH, discussed below

as part of the broad-spectrum antimicrobial program. All such anthrax antimicrobial programs are intended to address drug resistant anthrax as well.

Mid-Term (FY15-17)

Anthrax Vaccine

(T.A.15) Early-stage research for next-generation anthrax vaccines is in progress at NIH, investigating various technologies for temperature stabilization and alternative routes of delivery. Results from these preliminary studies should be available after FY15.

(T.A.16) BARDA will support expansion of domestic manufacturing capacity for the currently licensed anthrax vaccine, including validating new manufacturing processes, conducting additional non-clinical and clinical studies, and pursuing licensure of a new facility. *(T.A.17)* Concurrently, BARDA will continue the development of the existing rPA vaccine candidates in its pipeline, and build on NIH investments to advance a next-generation anthrax vaccine toward licensure through validating manufacturing processes and conducting non-clinical and clinical studies. It is anticipated that as a result of these activities, a next-generation anthrax vaccine may be available for procurement for the SNS during the FY15-17 timeframe. *(T.A.18)* In addition, BARDA will provide vaccine candidates with advanced development and manufacturing assistance from the CIADMs.

Anthrax Antitoxin

(T.A.19) BARDA will maintain investigational plans to collect clinical data in at-risk populations during mass-casualty events and develop communication and education programs for antitoxin products.

Anthrax Antimicrobials and Diagnostics

(T.A.20) The PHEMCE will support efforts to develop more rapid drug sensitivity assays for anthrax under the leadership of CDC, DHS, and DoD.

Long-Term (FY18 and beyond)

Anthrax Vaccine

NIH long-term research in this area will pursue the development of anthrax vaccines with PEP potential that provide enhancements to the currently available vaccine for more effective utilization in public health emergencies. Ultimately, the objective is an anthrax vaccine for PEP that is effective in one dose and produces a rapid onset of immunity, resulting in a substantially reduced requirement for the length and extent of antimicrobial PEP therapy.

BARDA will continue to support advanced development of next-generation anthrax vaccines, including use of non-clinical studies to evaluate efficacy. BARDA will also continue to support studies to evaluate vaccine with various adjuvants, establishment of master cell banks, and potential scale-up of manufacturing. In addition, BARDA will offer rPA active pharmaceutical ingredient to developers for enhancement studies under BARDA's Broad Agency Announcement (BAA). Finally, BARDA will continue to provide vaccine candidates with advanced development and manufacturing assistance from the CIADMs.

Anthrax Antitoxin

Research activities related to novel and simplified forms of antitoxins are underway at NIH and are expected to yield results in the long term. BARDA will support the advanced development of next-generation, small molecule antitoxins for treatment of anthrax as they become available. This will include efforts to ensure that appropriate animal models are available for advanced development.

Anthrax Antimicrobials and Diagnostics

NIH will support research into diagnostic platforms and the identification of biomarkers indicative of anthrax exposure to inform clinical decisions relative to antibiotic PEP administration. Additionally, NIH will support research into a more detailed characterization in the setting of symptomatic anthrax disease in order to guide clinical decisions regarding optimal antimicrobial therapy, as well as the need for additional antitoxin therapy.

The PHEMCE will support efforts to develop more rapid drug sensitivity assays for anthrax under the leadership of CDC, DHS, and DoD.

OTHER BACTERIAL THREATS

PHEMCE programmatic priorities for other bacterial threats include:

- Providing additional MCMs for the treatment and/or PEP of diseases caused by biological threat agents through discovery of novel targets that demonstrate effectiveness against drug-resistant variants and address bacterial agents for which an MTD has been made

- Revitalizing the pipeline of antimicrobial drugs to treat hospital- and community-acquired multi-drug resistant (MDR) bacterial infections for use in routine public health applications
- Establishing public-private partnerships to incentivize companies developing antimicrobials to both continue their commercial development and initiate development for biodefense indications.

Near-Term (FY12-14)

(T.OB.1) NIH maintains in vitro and animal model testing services for the infectious disease community, especially for those bacterial threats for which special handling is required (e.g., due to Select Agent status, Biosafety Level [BSL] 3 containment requirements, etc.). (T.OB.2) In addition, NIH will qualify animal efficacy models for anthrax, plague, and tularemia in support of PEP and treatment indications, through the FDA's animal model qualification process.

(T.OB.3) NIH will augment – beyond the recently approved plague datasets – antimicrobial efficacy datasets in support of clinical indications for anthrax, plague, and tularemia for off- patent antimicrobials in the SNS and/or in routine use. (T.OB.4) Additionally, NIH will support studies to inform utilization policy and response planning for these products.

(T.OB.5) BARDA will support the advanced research and development of novel antimicrobials and antiviral drugs for PEP and treatment of biological threat agents while addressing the threat of antimicrobial resistance in routine public health settings. (T.OB.6) BARDA also plans to develop animal models for testing MCMs against Burkholderia pseudomallei and Burkholderia mallei.

Mid-Term (FY15-17)

(T.OB.7) NIH will maintain antibiotic efficacy datasets for off-patent antimicrobials within the SNS, as well as for antimicrobials in common routine use. (T.OB.8) BARDA will initiate the testing of candidate products against Burkholderia pseudomallei and Burkholderia mallei.

Long-Term (FY18 and beyond)

BARDA will support late-stage development research activities in support of PEP and treatment of *Burkholderia* infections.

SMALLPOX

The PHEMCE smallpox programmatic priorities include:

- Maintaining an adequate stockpile of vaccines and VIG
- FDA licensure of Modified Vaccinia Ankara (MVA) vaccine, intended for use in at-risk populations
- Approval of two smallpox antivirals with different courses of action

Near-Term (FY12-14)

Smallpox Vaccine

Existing smallpox vaccines are mature. *(T.S.1)* In the near term, the PHEMCE will maintain sufficient quantities of smallpox vaccines in the SNS to provide a response capability to vaccinate every American during a smallpox emergency, if appropriate, including use of a vaccine for at-risk populations.

The PHEMCE will also publish the National Smallpox Vaccine Response Strategy, which will offer guidance on domestic vaccination strategies, as well as vaccine selection and prioritization for select subgroups, in an emergency triggered by a confirmed clinical case of smallpox. ASPR and CDC, working with FDA, will also focus on the development of a clinical utilization policy to describe the recommended emergency use of all currently stockpiled smallpox vaccines.

(T.S.2) CDC will focus on maintenance of the currently licensed smallpox vaccine, ACAM2000, and on the stockpile of VIG to treat adverse events resulting from smallpox vaccination. *(T.S.3)* BARDA will also continue development of a freeze-dried formulation of MVA to allow a longer shelf life and storage at higher temperatures in order to reduce lifecycle management costs.

Smallpox Antivirals and Diagnostics

Antivirals for the treatment of smallpox are in advanced development. *(T.S.4)* BARDA will deliver to the SNS a subset of the required treatment courses of the smallpox antivirals currently under contract, with full delivery being completed in the mid term.

(T.S.5) CDC will continue to support the development of IND protocols and/or pre-EUA packages for smallpox antivirals for regulatory review by FDA to allow for the stockpiling, distribution, dispensing, and utilization of these products in the event of an emergency. *(T.S.6)*

CDC will also conduct studies (including animal model studies) to inform the clinical use of these MCMs.

(T.S.7) In addition, CDC will continue to evaluate relevant diagnostic assays using both *in vitro* and *in vivo* systems to support FDA regulatory review and ultimately national use of these tests. These assays will include orthopoxvirus-generic and Variola-specific assays to be used in the Laboratory Response Network (LRN).

Mid- and Long-Term (FY15 and beyond)

Smallpox Vaccine

In the mid and long term, the PHEMCE will continue to maintain smallpox vaccines and VIG (as needed) in the SNS. *(T.S.8)* CDC will continue to work in coordination with the PHEMCE to project VIG needs based on demographic information and previous case history, and to identify research for informing improved VIG dosing.

(T.S.9) BARDA, working with CDC, will support activities to achieve FDA licensure for the MVA smallpox vaccine (intended for use in at-risk populations). *(T.S.10)* BARDA will provide technical support for the manufacture and acquisition of the MVA vaccine for at-risk populations. BARDA will also manage the transition from the present liquid-frozen form of the MVA smallpox vaccine to a freeze-dried formulation with superior lifecycle management properties. ASPR, CDC, and FDA will continue to work on the clinical guidance for smallpox vaccines.

Smallpox Antivirals

(T.S.11) NIH efforts focused on next-generation smallpox antivirals will support those products that emerge from the broad- spectrum antiviral program. Once those candidates have obtained FDA approval for other viral

indications, most likely via traditional Phase III safety and efficacy trials, NIH will pursue an orthopox clinical indication under the Animal Rule.

PANDEMIC INFLUENZA

The HHS PHEMCE pandemic influenza programmatic priorities include:

- Maintain the established comprehensive portfolio approach to develop, acquire, and build an infrastructure for a broad array of MCMs to respond to pandemic influenza – including vaccines, therapeutics, diagnostics, and non-pharmaceutical countermeasures
- Build and sustain a domestic manufacturing capacity
- Address various aspects of MCM utilization for pandemic influenza and develop and distribute communication and educational materials before and/or during an influenza pandemic
- Develop a novel antigen or "universal" flu vaccine that will eliminate the need for annual modifications to the influenza vaccine or annual boosters

Near-term (FY12-14)[69]

Influenza Antigen-Sparing Technology

(T.PI.1) Beginning in the near term and extending into the mid term, NIH and BARDA will jointly support a wide portfolio of new and ongoing adjuvant discovery, development, and testing activities. The goal is to provide antigen-sparing benefits (i.e., decreased amount of viral hemagglutinin antigen needed to provide immunity), broad heterosubtypic immunity (i.e., protection against multiple virus variants), and prime-boost effects (i.e., one dose may be sufficient instead of two or more) for influenza vaccines.

Communications and Response Planning

(T.PI.2) Beginning in the near term and extending over five years, CDC will ensure that operational plans for pandemic influenza communication are updated, exercised, evaluated, and improved to facilitate effective communication strategies. Furthermore, CDC will develop mechanisms to further integrate social media and other communication tools into preparedness activities. CDC will also improve and share public health

emergency messages, including translated and culturally appropriate materials for non-English- speaking communities across the U.S., and increase the capacity for developing plain language and easily understood materials for public audiences. In addition, CDC will (1) develop procedures to ensure that information in future pandemics is provided in accessible and alternative formats; (2) refine and implement partnership strategies to improve communication with hard-to-reach and at-risk populations; (3) use partnerships and other information dissemination channels to effectively reach and inform clinicians regarding CDC's policies, guidelines, and recommendations related to pandemic influenza MCMs; and (4) develop an approach, definitions, tools and models for a risk communication response plan.

Influenza Vaccine Stockpiles

(T.PI.3) BARDA will maintain and update the existing stockpile of novel influenza virus and pre-pandemic vaccines and adjuvants as needed. Recognizing the continuous evolution of the H5N1 viruses, stockpile purchases will be balanced among clade 1 and clade 2 antigenic virus strains and may evolve to address other novel influenza virus threats as warranted.

(T.PI.4) CDC, working with BARDA and FDA, will develop rapid methods to produce candidate vaccine viruses that allow accelerated production of vaccine lots for eventual fill and finish by manufacturers. In addition, in collaboration with BARDA and FDA, CDC will complete work on the development of rapid laboratory methods to expedite testing to determine the antigen content of influenza vaccine bulk material and enable vaccine formulation prior to product fill and finish.

Influenza Vaccine Development

(T.PI.5) NIH is focusing on a wide array of novel viral antigen and universal influenza vaccine concepts, with several candidates entering preclinical development over the next several years. *(T.PI.6)* NIH is also developing a repository of required influenza-related reagents to support universal influenza vaccine development. *(T.PI.7)* In addition, NIH is working closely with the FDA to develop and refine additional assays to support future vaccine development efforts.

Cell- and recombinant-based influenza vaccine development is a key element in the PHEMCE intermediate and long-term pandemic influenza preparedness strategy in order to provide adequate domestic vaccine manufacturing surge capacity. *(T.PI.8)* BARDA is supporting the advanced development of and pursuit of FDA licensure for cell-based influenza vaccines, as well as *(T.PI.9)* the development of novel recombinant vaccine candidates for both pandemic and seasonal influenza through Phase II clinical trials, in this timeframe. *(T.PI.10)* As novel viral antigen or universal influenza vaccine candidates are developed through proof-of-concept Phase I clinical trials, BARDA will support the advanced development of these candidates toward licensed products.

(T.PI.11) CDC will continue refining the Influenza Risk Assessment Tool (IRAT). The IRAT was developed by CDC and federal, non-federal, international, public health, and academic influenza experts as an evaluation tool to measure the potential pandemic risk posed by influenza A viruses currently circulating in animals but not yet in humans. The tool allows designated influenza subject matter experts to consider ten scientific criteria measuring the potential pandemic risk posed by particular viral strains, and thereby assists BARDA and the federal government in prioritizing which viruses should become vaccine virus candidates and possibly produced as vaccines for the pandemic influenza vaccine stockpile.

Influenza Antivirals

(T.PI.12) NIH will support post-Phase IIa development of an influenza broad-spectrum therapeutic with multi-functional potential. NIH will also develop both small molecule drugs and monoclonal antibodies as broad-spectrum influenza therapeutics. These therapeutics will initially be developed as treatments, with the potential for prophylactic use in future, especially in those individuals for whom vaccine responses are poor.

(T.PI.13) BARDA will support development of existing neuraminidase inhibitor drugs and host-targeted antiviral drug candidates, as well as new combination therapies, monoclonal antibody therapies, and new classes of influenza antiviral drugs.

(T.PI.14) CDC will expand surveillance for antiviral susceptibility. *(T.PI.15)* PHEMCE partners, including CDC, NIH, BARDA, and FDA will review and evaluate the potential benefits and disadvantages of different antiviral use strategies, and reassess the quantity and composition of antiviral stockpiles by various levels of government and other partners, taking fiscal constraints and manufacturing capacity into account. *(T.PI.16)* CDC will also develop new plans for influenza antiviral distribution and dispensing.

Influenza Diagnostics

(T.PI.17) NIH will sequence genomic data for influenza viral isolates to support current and future diagnostics efforts. In addition, NIH will continue to add representative influenza viral isolates to NIH's National Institute of Allergy and Infectious Diseases (NIAID) Biodefense and Emerging Infections (BEI) Research Resources Repository in order to make strains available for developing next-generation diagnostic tests.

(T.PI.18) CDC will seek FDA clearance for a new test to distinguish the two major lineages of Influenza B and to improve rapid genetic sequencing for surveillance of influenza. CDC will also work to gain FDA clearance for the use of alternative enzymes in the previously cleared CDC laboratory diagnostic kit, which diagnoses human infections with seasonal influenza viruses and novel influenza A viruses with pandemic potential. *(T.PI.19)* CDC will also develop and provide timely guidance and support to clinicians on using improved diagnostic testing for disease management and treatment.

(T.PI.20) BARDA will continue the development of point-of-care diagnostic devices for detection of influenza and other respiratory pathogens, including intentional biological threat agents. *(T.PI.21)* CDC and BARDA will commence development of new sequencing-based diagnostic assays and prototype device development for detection of influenza viruses and other respiratory pathogens.

Influenza Respiratory Protective Devices

(T.PI.22) To address pandemic influenza in particular, in the near-term CDC and BARDA will develop systems to monitor potential shortages of respiratory protective devices (RPDs) during an influenza pandemic.

Mid-Term (FY15-17)

Communications and Response Planning

(T.PI.23) CDC will refine and expand the use of immunization information systems among all providers, including non-traditional providers.

Influenza Vaccine Stockpiles

(T.PI.24) CDC will seek to increase the percentage of persons receiving annual influenza vaccinations.[70] *(T.PI.25)* CDC will also work with federal and SLTT partners to implement guidance developed by the USG for situations in which limited vaccine availability requires targeted vaccination of

persons with high-risk conditions. *(T.PI.26)* BARDA will maintain and adjust novel influenza virus and pre-pandemic influenza vaccine stockpiles as warranted.

Influenza Vaccine Development

(T.PI.27) NIH anticipates moving several universal influenza vaccine candidates into early-phase human clinical testing to provide clinical proof-of-concept for the validity of immunogenicity with broad cross-protective immunity to disparate influenza strains. *(T.PI.28)* BARDA will support at least one novel viral antigen or universal vaccine candidate expected to be evaluated in Phase II clinical studies in the mid term.

(T.PI.29) BARDA will continue support for the advanced development of recombinant influenza vaccine candidates that are anticipated to complete Phase III clinical studies, followed by BLA filings for licensure, in this timeframe.

Influenza Antivirals

(T.PI.30) BARDA will support advanced development of at least two drugs with novel mechanism(s) of action through Phase III clinical studies; two drugs are expected to be approved for use in the U.S.

Influenza Diagnostics

(T.PI.31) CDC will ensure implementation of laboratory reference diagnostics for influenza at public health laboratories and refine the methods by which specimens are tested for surveillance purposes. Expansion of capacity to rapidly detect novel influenza viruses and emerging antiviral resistance is also planned. In addition, CDC will improve the timeliness and accuracy of laboratory assays for measuring influenza immunity. *(T.PI.32)* Finally, CDC and BARDA will continue support of the development of sequencing-based diagnostic assays and prototype device development for detection of influenza viruses and other respiratory pathogens.

Long-term (FY18 and beyond)

Influenza Vaccine Stockpiles

BARDA will maintain and update the pre-pandemic stockpile as needed to maintain preparedness. When universal influenza vaccines are licensed, the PHEMCE will reexamine the utility of existing pre-pandemic stockpiles.

CDC will work to refine policies and plans related to pre-pandemic vaccine distribution modalities (e.g., pre-pandemic vaccine allocation guidance, utilization strategies, stockpiling goals, and communications plans). This effort will focus on the refinement of the pandemic vaccine prioritization strategy and implementation plans as necessary, including communication plans. In coordination with FDA, CDC will also conduct influenza vaccine safety studies in at-risk populations (e.g., pregnant women), and explore opportunities to improve awareness of vaccine adverse events and increase reporting to the Vaccine Adverse Event Reporting System (VAERS) by clinicians and other vaccine providers.

Influenza Vaccine Development

NIH is focusing on a wide array of universal influenza vaccine concepts, with several candidates entering preclinical development over the next several years. NIH is also developing a repository of required influenza-related reagents to support universal influenza vaccine development. In addition, NIH is working closely with the FDA to develop and refine additional assays, including sterility and potency testing, to support future vaccine development efforts.

BARDA will continue support of novel viral antigen or universal influenza vaccine candidate(s) through advanced development towards licensure.

Influenza Antivirals

In this time frame, it is anticipated that at least four additional antiviral drugs will be approved for use in the U.S., including the two existing drugs in development under a BARDA contract, and two new drugs that will be under contract in the near term.

OTHER VIRAL THREATS

For emerging infectious diseases, viral agents remain a dominant source of likely novel outbreaks. PHEMCE programmatic priorities for other viral threats include:

- Addressing existing viral threats
- Strengthening the capability to respond to emerging viral threats through a broad-spectrum antiviral program

Near-Term (FY12-14)

(T.OV.1) NIH is supporting research into therapeutic candidates for broad-spectrum antiviral treatments. In addition, NIH will offer in vitro and in vivo screening of newly discovered candidates. Initial targeted clinical indications include influenza, as well as certain viral hemorrhagic fevers. NIH will also continue its lead role in a USG-wide interagency working group developing specific reagents, assays, and animal efficacy models to support filovirus vaccine and therapeutic MCM approval.

Mid-Term (FY15-17)

(T.OV.2) NIH anticipates moving broad-spectrum antiviral candidates into clinical testing in this time frame. In addition, it will undertake animal efficacy model studies to validate these agents' broad-spectrum activity and examine their potential to replace existing stockpiled MCMs once they gain approval. (T.OV.3) BARDA will expand platform programs with the potential to address more threats, such as the filoviruses. (T.OV.4) BARDA also plans to support expanded formulations of existing antiviral drugs.

Long-Term (FY18 and beyond)

BARDA expects to diversify its portfolio to accommodate innovation while balancing portfolio risk and ensuring that at-risk population needs are addressed. Mid- to late-stage development activities for a filovirus therapeutic are anticipated to require continued support by BARDA.

BOTULISM

PHEMCE botulism programmatic priorities include:

- Establishing and maintaining a long-term supply of heptavalent botulism antitoxin
- Developing next-generation botulism therapeutics that offer more safe and effective treatment, as well as reduced manufacturing and storage costs

- Transitioning to a sustainable platform for long-term production

Near-Term (FY12-14)

(T.B.1) BARDA will support pursuit of FDA licensure of the equine-derived, heptavalent botulism antitoxin product. A pre-EUA package for this product was prepared by CDC and submitted to the FDA, and the Biologics License Application (BLA) for its licensure was submitted in FY12.

(T.B.2) CDC will continue to collect data on the heptavalent antitoxin's safety to inform use of this product. These data will also inform the USG botulism response plan. CDC has also developed and validated both botulinum toxin detection (enzyme-linked immunosorbent assay and mass spectrometry) applications and botulinum toxin gene (real time polymerase chain reaction) in vitro detection methods to confirm botulism in symptomatic persons.

(T.B.3) NIH will continue to evaluate a collection of next-generation botulism antitoxin monoclonal antibodies. A botulism serotype A cocktail is undergoing Phase I trials, while a botulism serotype B&E combination is in advanced preclinical evaluation. Serotypes C&D have recently entered initial preclinical testing, while serotype F&G candidates are still being evaluated.

Mid- and Long-Term (FY15 and beyond)

(T.B.4) BARDA will support studies on the use of the heptavalent product in at-risk populations, as well as communication and education programs on effective utilization of this MCM.

(T.B.5) Presuming successful testing of the next-generation serotype A and serotype B&E monoclonal antibody cocktails, serotypes A, B, & E will be combined into one product by NIH to investigate an MCM that would address more than 95% of naturally occurring botulism, as well as be appropriate for botulism cases in infants. (T.B.6) BARDA will support the advanced development of these next-generation products as they become eligible for transition from NIH.

RADIOLOGICAL AND NUCLEAR THREATS

PHEMCE programmatic priorities for radiological and nuclear threats include:

- Elucidating mechanisms of radiation injury at the system, organ, cell, and molecular levels, with special focus on the hematopoietic, gastrointestinal, immune, pulmonary, renal, skin, and nervous systems
- Identifying and characterizing MCM approaches to minimize the short- and long-term adverse health effects of radiation exposure, including cytokines, growth factors, antiapoptotics, anti-inflammatory agents, and antioxidant candidates, as well as products with other novel mechanisms of action
- Emphasizing candidates that have routine medical/clinical indications and can be administered effectively under current or anticipated CONOPs
- Developing definitive-care treatments for thermal burns, as well as providing incentives, through public-private partnerships, for companies developing thermal burn and other nuclear and radiological exposure treatments to continue commercial development while meeting civilian emergency preparedness requirements

Near-Term (FY12-14)

Medical Countermeasures for Acute Radiation Syndrome (ARS) and the Delayed Effects of Acute Radiation Exposure (DEARE)

NIH has identified more than 75 candidate MCMs in the early discovery phase for hematopoietic ARS. NIH has also identified more than fifteen candidates in the early discovery phase for gastrointestinal ARS and more than five candidates in the early discovery phase for the treatment of pulmonary radiation injuries. *(T.RN.1)* These candidates will continue to be evaluated and developed toward IND submission. Successful candidates will be identified that can move forward to BARDA for potential advanced development.

(T.RN.2) BARDA will support evaluation of a number of commercial drugs for repurposing to enable use in the treatment of exposure to radiological and nuclear agents, ensuring that at-risk population needs are considered. *(T.RN.3)* BARDA will also support the advanced research and development of novel compounds for PEP and treatment of exposure to radiological and nuclear threats. It is anticipated that a subset of the required treatment courses of antineutropenic colony-stimulating factors will be shipped to the SNS in the near term.

Thermal Burn Therapeutics

(T.RN.4) BARDA will assess results from the current proof-of-concept studies for promising candidates for thermal burn injuries and continue to support the development of thermal burn definitive care products.

Decorporation and Blocking Agents

(T.RN.5) NIH will continue to focus support for the development of oral formulations of actinide decorporation agents, as well as for the identification and development of new radionuclide decorporation and blocking agents that prevent uptake and/or increase the elimination of internal contamination with a range of radionuclides.

(T.RN.6) BARDA will continue to fund projects to support advanced research and development of Prussian blue formulations appropriate for children under the age of two years.

Mid-Term (FY15-FY17)

Medical Countermeasures for Acute Radiation Syndrome (ARS) and the Delayed Effects of Acute Radiation Exposure (DEARE)

NIH will continue to evaluate additional candidates for hematopoietic ARS, gastrointestinal ARS and pulmonary radiation injuries in rodent and non-human primate animal models, and in INDenabling studies. Successful candidates will be identified that can move forward to BARDA for potential advanced development. *(T.RN.7)* Rodent and non-human primate animal models are being further developed and will be qualified for pivotal animal efficacy studies. *(T.RN.8)* CDC and ASPR, working closely other PHEMCE partners, will finalize clinical guidance for MCMs to address radiation-induced neutropenia.

Long-Term (FY18 and beyond)

In the long term, BARDA will place more emphasis upon achieving regulatory approval of MCMs for use in treating injuries from radiation exposure.

Medical Countermeasures for Acute Radiation Syndrome (ARS) and the Delayed Effects of Acute Radiation Exposure (DEARE)

BARDA will continue acquisition of anti-neutropenic products for the SNS as necessary. Using appropriate animal models, BARDA will support studies to obtain additional data to support preEUA applications and ultimately regulatory approval for these products.

Decorporation and Blocking Agents

BARDA will monitor programs under development at NIH to determine if and when they may be eligible for transition to BARDA.

CHEMICAL THREATS

The HHS PHEMCE chemical programmatic priorities include:

- Developing *in vitro* and animal models for efficacy screening of novel therapeutics
- Developing MCMs for the treatment of injuries caused by exposure to chemical threats, with an emphasis on products that can be administered effectively under current or anticipated CONOPs
- Maintaining public-private partnerships with companies developing chemical agent treatments

Near- and Mid-Term (FY12-17)

(T.C.1) NIH is supporting investments against classical chemical agents (e.g., nerve agents and vesicants), and toxic industrial chemicals (TICs). Included are compounds that can damage the nervous system, respiratory tract, skin and mucous membranes, and other organs. NIH also supports investments in promising anticonvulsants, such as midazolam, a potential replacement for diazepam for the treatment of nerve agent-induced seizures. Other research thrusts include more effective and more easily administered MCMs against cyanide.

(T.C.2) BARDA will continue to support the advanced research and development of novel compounds for treatment or PEP following exposure to chemical agents, including patient decontamination solutions for use on intact or injured human skin, with improved efficacy over soap and water.[71] (T.C.3)

BARDA will also evaluate commercially available drugs using animal models to determine if their approved use can be expanded to the treatment of chemical exposures. (T.C.4) In addition, BARDA will support the regulatory approval process for products treating injuries due to exposure to chemical agents.

Long-Term (FY18 and beyond)

This will include an emphasis on TIC exposures, such as industrial chemicals and pesticides. Planned activities include: (1) integrating research of potential products into evolving standards of emergency care; (2) assessing products already approved/licensed/cleared for use in the U.S. for applicability to chemical casualty care; (3) assessing products from military applications for civilian use; and (4) developing and/or improving medical diagnostic tests and assays to detect the presence of specific chemicals or their metabolites in bodily fluids.

BARDA will support the advanced research and development of novel compounds for PEP and treatment following exposure to chemical agents. Emphasis will be placed on achieving regulatory approval of products for use in treating injuries due to chemical agent exposures. BARDA will also support the potential for repurposing commercial products approved/licensed/cleared for other uses for potential use as treatments for exposure to chemical agents.

SUMMARY OF THREAT-BASED APPROACHES

The PHEMCE focus on threat-specific needs will continue to be a high priority approach over the next five years. Successful MCM development since the *2007 PHEMCE Strategy* and *Implementation Plan* has led to procurement of critical products for the SNS. However, there is still a significant need to incorporate products that cover the full spectrum of threats and to make improvements in currently held products (e.g., lower lifecycle costs, accelerate time to availability, improve operational performance, enhance ability to meet at-risk population needs). In the near term, efforts are being focused on completing investments made in areas of the highest-priority threats, while mid- and long-term efforts will focus on moving toward broader, multi-functional, and platform technologies to satisfy the need for agile responses that will still be effective against the highest-priority threats.

SECTION 4: CAPABILITIES-BASED APPROACHES

The PHEMCE is evolving from programs focused on rapidly developing and acquiring medical products critical for bolstering preparedness, to programs that will provide more flexible and sustainable capabilities over the long term. This is best reflected in the PHEMCE's promotion of technologies that have more than one application, and/or of infrastructures that can be rapidly adjusted to surge to new demands and respond to new threats. This evolution is highly dependent on early-stage research and early identification of biotechnologies that may already be applied in routine product development. NIH programs on platform technologies and broad-spectrum approaches are thus key to fueling this early pipeline. Similarly, efforts underway at BARDA are critical in advancing the nation's capability to build and sustain a flexible manufacturing and development infrastructure, as well as in identifying products that may be repurposed or altered to meet PHEMCE needs. In addition to the many cross-cutting capabilities described in Section 1 with respect to the strategic goals and objectives they address, this section highlights several specific examples of these capabilities-based approaches.

CBRN DIAGNOSTICS

PHEMCE programmatic priorities for CBRN diagnostics include:

- Developing both high-throughput and point-of-care (POC) diagnostics that will inform the use of MCMs for the treatment of conditions or diseases caused by radiological agents, biological pathogens, or chemical agents/toxins
- Developing platform technologies that offer the capacity for a multiplexed capability, so that as additional threats are encountered, they can be seamlessly integrated into extant systems
- Developing and advancing diagnostic policies to prevent, detect, and control public health security threats from CBRN agents.

Near-Term (FY12-14)

(C.D.1) NIH will initiate funding for the development of biological agent diagnostic systems, chemical agent diagnostic systems, and systems to identify and characterize unknown threats, including development of assays and instrumentation to address PHEMCE requirements for high-throughput and POC usage. (C.D.2) NIH will also work in conjunction with FDA to define alternative methodologies for the generation of requisite datasets for specific threat agents for which traditional clinical specimens are insufficient to support approval.

(C.D.3) BARDA will fund development of biodosimetry assays and devices and integrate the development of high-throughput biodosimetry assays with commercial off-the-shelf (COTS) diagnostic instrumentation to achieve high-throughput biodosimetry diagnostic systems. (C.D.4) BARDA will also work closely with interagency partners to develop an appropriate stockpiling strategy for each product.

Mid-Term (FY15-17)

(C.D.5) NIH will develop reference profile panels of threat agents that will support generation of requisite datasets required for licensure of a next-generation diagnostic platform. (C.D.6) BARDA will fund the development, implementation, agency approval, manufacturing preparation, and appropriate stockpiling strategy implementation for biodosimetry diagnostic systems for use in POC and high-throughput laboratory settings using clinical samples.

(C.D.7) CDC will develop and validate additional radionuclide bioassay diagnostic tests to allow rapid detection and measurement of radionuclides in clinical specimens. The goal is to develop a suite of assays capable of rapidly detecting the radionuclides identified by DHS as most likely to be used in radiological terrorism. These assays can be used to identify who was internally contaminated in an incident, and to assess the need for, and efficacy of, decorporation therapy.

Long-Term (FY18 and beyond)

In the long term, BARDA will support activities that include development, implementation, agency approval, manufacturing preparation, and appropriate stockpiling for CBRN diagnostic systems, including both assays and instrumentation, for identifying and characterizing unknown threats in both high-throughput and POC systems.

NON-PHARMACEUTICAL MEDICAL COUNTERMEASURES

Near-Term (FY12-14)

(C.NP.1) CDC certifies respiratory protective devices (RPDs) and maintains a "Trusted Sources Webpage" so that informed RPD selection decisions can be made.[72] CDC will continue to focus research on three areas: protecting emergency medical technicians (EMT) in ambulances; development of expedient isolation methods; and development of improved negative pressure isolation room designs.

(C.NP.2) To ensure preparedness for effective use of RPDs, CDC will encourage RPD manufacturers to pursue both National Institute for Occupational Safety and Health (NIOSH) certification and FDA clearance to ensure an ample supply of FDA-cleared N95 respirators. (C.NP.3) In addition, CDC will strengthen RPD design, use, testing, and certification for the occupational setting. (C.NP.4)

The CDC will also reassess the quantity and composition of respirator stockpiles for pandemic influenza and other threats, taking fiscal constraints into account, to determine whether the stockpiling of respirators in the SNS should be continued.

If so, the PHEMCE will develop respirator stockpiling requirements. (C.NP.5) In addition, beginning in the near-term and extending beyond 2017, CDC will conduct research to better understand influenza transmission, clarify when surgical masks are sufficient, and determine when the use of N95 respirators or other devices may be more appropriate.

(C.NP.6) The PHEMCE will develop an all-hazards ventilator assessment that will define both the quantities of ventilators for stockpiling and the desired device attributes[73] for effectively responding to a range of lung injuries associated with different threat agents. This assessment will incorporate an analysis of the number of trained personnel in the U.S. who are capable of providing mechanical ventilation oversight and are likely to be available when needed in an emergency.

The analysis will help identify whether there is likely to be a shortage of ventilator-trained personnel during a mass-casualty public health emergency, and review options for minimizing that shortage. Finally, since mechanical ventilators may be a scarce resource during a mass-casualty incident, the assessment will review existing strategies for ethical allocation of ventilators during a public health emergency.

(C.NP.7) A national planning guidance for conducting mass patient decontamination in a chemical incident, an effort co-led by HHS and DHS, will be published in the near term. *(C.NP.8)* HHS and DHS will then begin work with appropriate organizations to integrate the planning guidance into emergency response training curricula. *(C.NP.9)* BARDA will initiate a research program to address critical knowledge gaps in the subject of patient decontamination.

Mid-Term (FY15-17)

(C.NP.10) CDC will work with standard-setting organizations to incorporate healthcare worker respiratory protective equipment (RPE) research project findings on improving respirator compliance, comfort, and tolerability into industry and consensus standards. Similar efforts will be undertaken with the ambulance, expedient isolation, and negative pressure isolation research project findings.

(C.NP.11) CDC will reassess strategies for distributing SNS ventilators to the states to help ensure federal assets will be used equitably; develop systems to monitor the safety, effectiveness, and shortages of RPDs after deployment; and develop and/or revise relevant RPD use/reuse guidance and policies.

CENTERS FOR INNOVATION IN ADVANCED DEVELOPMENT AND MANUFACTURING

PHEMCE programmatic priorities for the Centers for Innovation in Advanced Development and Manufacturing (CIADMs or centers) include:

- Expanding the nation's domestic ability to respond to bioterrorism threats, pandemic influenza, and other epidemics by providing experienced biopharmaceutical developers to aid biotech innovators, resulting in a more robust, timely, and successful product development pipeline and stockpile
- Incorporating innovative technologies that will provide a more efficient model for MCM product development relative to cost and time
- Providing domestic manufacturing surge capacity for pandemic influenza vaccine[74]

Near-Term (FY12-14)

(C.CIADM.1) BARDA will support the initial planning and engineering activities related to the construction of critical infrastructure within the CIADMs. It is anticipated that these centers will have limited capability to provide certain advanced development and manufacturing core services during this time frame, if required by the USG. The centers will also be initiating the activities required for the licensing of a pandemic influenza vaccine candidate, including in-licensing as needed, and process development related to the eventual technology transfer of the candidate into the facility. *(C.CIADM.2)* BARDA, along with its PHEMCE partners, will establish the CIADM governance structure.

Mid-Term (FY15-17)

(C.CIADM.3) BARDA will support the construction and qualification phases of the establishment of new critical infrastructure within the CIADMs. (C.CIADM.4) BARDA will also support, through the CIADM governance board, the issuance, evaluation, and contract award for advanced development and manufacturing core services as programs flow from HHS and DoD programs.

Long-Term (FY18 and beyond)

BARDA will support the licensure of the pandemic influenza vaccine candidates in the CIADMs and will provide for the appropriate framework to maintain a state of readiness in the event of a pandemic or other national public health emergency.

The centers will be assisting small biotech companies with technology, regulatory affairs, quality systems, and manufacturing expertise to reach the goal of a licensed and readily available product for public and private use. Center academic partners will offer advanced training for the next generation of biotechnology workers. The centers will continue to support advanced development of other MCMs as they are transitioned from BARDA and DoD early development programs.

CROSS-CUTTING CAPABILITIES

The PHEMCE has developed a range of capabilities that could address multiple potential national health security threats, as well as the multiple goals and objectives identified in the *2012 PHEMCE Strategy*. This subsection summarizes some of these cross-cutting capabilities; many of these are described in greater detail in Section 1 with respect to the strategic goals and objectives they address.

PHEMCE programmatic priorities for Product Development Core Services include:

- If authorized by Congress, establishing the Medical Countermeasures Strategic Investor to provide venture capital funding and services to firms developing commercially viable products that address biodefense requirements
- Developing a suite of preclinical and advanced development core service capabilities to improve the efficiency of public-private partnerships in delivering needed medical countermeasures
- Qualifying an array of animal models to support product development under the Animal Rule
- Building and maintaining a world-class workforce of subject matter experts in the management of clinical trials, regulatory and quality affairs, pharmacology and toxicology, manufacturing and bioprocessing, analytic decision support, and modeling

As described in greater detail under Goals 1 and 2, NIH and BARDA provide a range of core services in support of MCM development and manufacturing. In the near term, BARDA will establish a CRO Network and *(C.CC.1)* Fill-Finish Network (FFN) to support, respectively, the performance of needed or urgent clinical trials and the filling and finishing of vaccines and biological therapeutics in circumstances where additional capacity is required. *(C.CC.2)* NIH will continue to maintain its Vaccine and Treatment Evaluation Units (VTEUs) for vaccine testing capacity during clinical trials in support of public health emergencies. *(C.CC.3)* If authorized by Congress, BARDA will establish the Medical Countermeasures Strategic Investor (MCMSI) and MCMSI Interface Office (MIO).

BARDA, in conjunction with NIH, will support the development of new animal models for burkholderia, tularemia, ARS, and other material threats as needed. *(C.CC.4)* BARDA will also establish a Visualization Hub to provide analytic decision support and access to real-time modeling capabilities to senior decision makers within ASPR and the PHEMCE. BARDA will continue to adapt its business model and provision of core services to complement the capabilities and strengths of its private sector partners, reducing redundant efforts and streamlining the product development pathway. NIH will continue to manage the CAP, which is designed to accelerate development of promising MCMs.

(C.CC.5) In the mid term, NIH, BARDA, and FDA will expand the number of qualified animal models, focusing on models for the highest-priority threats and those needed for maturing product development initiatives. *(C.CC.6)* The MCMSI will expand its portfolio of investments based on strategic requirements developed by the MIO in consultation with PHEMCE partners and in accordance with available resources. BARDA will fully integrate the provision of core services into its public-private partnerships, adapting increasingly flexible models of partnership to expedite product development and facilitate long-term strategic relationships. *(C.CC.7)* NIH's infrastructure services will continue to provide appropriate *in vitro* and *in vivo* testing for candidate countermeasures, especially those requiring adequate biocontainment facilities, as well as product-specific services, in support of overall anti-infective development capabilities.

FDA plays a critical role in supporting the MCM mission from discovery through development to deployment and use. As described under Goal 2, FDA works with PHEMCE partners to identify and resolve regulatory and scientific challenges that impede MCM development and use across all PHEMCE priorities. For example, FDA – through its MCMi – has established multidisciplinary Public Health and Security Action Teams to identify and help resolve regulatory and scientific challenges for high-priority MCMs and related technologies; an MCM Regulatory Science Program to build the science base necessary to support MCM development and regulatory assessment; and a policy team that works to ensure that FDA laws, regulations, and policies adequately support MCM development, distribution, and use. FDA also works directly with both individual product developers and the MCM development community to clarify regulatory requirements and provide scientific and technical expert review of MCM product applications, with the ultimate goal of approving/licensing/clearing MCMs. In addition, FDA fosters preparedness and effective, timely responses to public health emergencies with MCMs that are available but not yet FDA-approved for the intended use through a variety of regulatory mechanisms that allow for emergency use of such products.

CDC maintains several cross-cutting capabilities that can be drawn upon to help provide medical countermeasures in a timely manner and reduce the adverse health impacts during an emergency. *(C.CC.8)* CDC's core laboratory science, epidemiology, and surveillance functions provide public health authorities with timely, accurate, and interpretable information that enables health officials to make informed decisions – such as placement and use of MCMs, and social distancing measures – needed for saving lives and protecting the public.

(C.CC.9) Within CDC there is a core laboratory capacity to detect, identify, confirm, and quantify the vast majority of the high-priority biological, chemical and radiological threat agents. *(C.CC.10)* In addition, CDC manages the Laboratory Response Network (LRN), a group of local, state, federal and international laboratories with unique testing capabilities for detecting high-priority biological and chemical threat agents. LRN labs play a critical role in our nation's ability to detect, characterize, and communicate confirmed threat agents.

(C.CC.11) CDC also supports some 280 surveillance-related activities to monitor and assess the population's health, including BioSense 2.0, ILINet, and PulseNet, which may help authorities detect and characterize (or confirm) an attack. In addition, CDC supports the development, evaluation, and improvement of state and local capabilities for MCM distribution and dispensing through programs providing guidance, training, exercise, and evaluation for MCM preparedness and response functions.

Finally, the DSNS maintains partnerships for priority access to ground and air transportation to deliver medicines and supplies for state and local emergency response. *(C.CC.12)* Similarly, CDC's Vaccines for Children (VFC) infrastructure offers a mechanism for ordering and shipping routine childhood vaccines as well as pandemic influenza vaccine to health departments and other vaccine providers in the event of a disease outbreak.

The DoD cross-cutting initiatives that support the PHEMCE include laboratory facilities located both within and outside the contiguous U.S., *(C.CC.13)* and a soon-to-be-established MCM advanced development and manufacturing facility. The facility, when fully established, will be able to work cooperatively with analogous facilities established by HHS. Current DoD laboratory capabilities include dedicated space to conduct studies at all biological safety levels; facilitate the discovery and early development of vaccines, therapeutics, and diagnostics and the associated relevant animal models for the evaluation of new MCMs; and provide the infrastructure and personnel to characterize emerging chemical and biological threats.

(C.CC.14) The DoD has embarked on a long-term stewardship effort to maintain its MCM capabilities and is currently refurbishing its chemical and biological flagship laboratories.

These efforts, critical to DoD, are also integral to the nation by providing a sustained set of assets and scientific expertise necessary for MCM development. Specifically, the DoD is establishing a dedicated biological safety level 4 laboratory capable of conducting tests that meet GLP requirements and evaluation of MCMs, and is also investing in state of the art laboratory facilities.

The overall cooperative efforts between HHS and DoD with regard to advanced development and manufacturing provide an agile and responsive capacity for the nation to manufacture MCMs. *(C.CC.15)* Along with MCM development, the DoD continues to develop programs such as biosurveillance and support of diagnostics to aid the interagency in the use of MCMs to protect the population.

SUMMARY OF CAPABILITIES-BASED APPROACHES

The PHEMCE has started to direct its investments, where possible, from products, platforms or approaches that address single threats toward capabilities that offer a greater likelihood of broad-spectrum or multi-functional approaches that address more than one threat. The potential side benefits of this approach include platforms and products that may have greater commercial viability for public health or routine medical needs, as well as adaptation of commercial products for PHEMCE-specific needs. Key concepts in the evolution of this approach have included a focus on rapid scale-up of development times for products and on creative means for more rapidly procuring products.

Near-term commitments in this process include the creation of core services and rapid-scale up production of biologics, as represented by the CIADMs. Mid-term and long-term efforts are represented by NIH and DoD efforts to identify promising technologies that offer novel broad-spectrum approaches.

CONCLUSION

This *2012 PHEMCE Implementation Plan* identifies the top priorities and projected timelines for MCM research, development, acquisition, stockpiling, distribution, dispensing, and monitoring programs, as well as initiatives that HHS has determined, in collaboration with interagency partners throughout the PHEMCE, will make the best use of available resources to improve public health emergency preparedness and advance national health security.

The PHEMCE will identify projected milestones and timelines for these priorities, and ASPR will establish the necessary management processes and tools to track, monitor, and evaluate their execution. Periodic updates will be provided through the PHEMCE governance structure.

This tracking system will facilitate accountability, foster coordination, and identify and address potential challenges in pursuit of these important goals and objectives. It is anticipated that the *PHEMCE Strategy* and *Implementation Plan* will be reviewed and updated every five years or more frequently if needed.

APPENDIX 1. ACRONYMS

ACF	Administration for Children and Families
ADM	Advanced Development and Manufacturing
AMT	Anthrax Management Team (BARDA, CDC)
ARS	Acute Radiation Syndrome
ASPR	Assistant Secretary for Preparedness and Response
BARDA	Biomedical Advanced Research and Development Authority
BAA	Broad Agency Announcement
BEI	Biodefense and Emerging Infections
BLA	Biologics License Application
BSA	Broad Spectrum Antimicrobial
BSC	Board of Scientific Counselors (CDC)
BSL	Biosafety Level
CAP	Concept Acceleration Program (NIH)
CBER	Center for Biologics Evaluation and Research (FDA)
CBRN	Chemical, Biological, Radiological, and Nuclear
CDC	Centers for Disease Control and Prevention
CHILD	Children's HHS Interagency Leadership on Disasters
CDER	Center for Drug Evaluation and Research (FDA)
CDRH	Center for Devices and Radiological Health (FDA)
CIADMs	Centers for Innovation in Advanced Development and Manufacturing
CONOPs	Concepts of Operations

COTS	Commercial Off-The-Shelf
CRO	Contract Research Organization
DDT	Drug Development Tool
DEARE	Delayed Effects of Radiation Exposure
DHS	Department of Homeland Security
DLG	Disaster Leadership Group (ASPR)
DoD	Department of Defense
DSNS	Division of Strategic National Stockpile (CDC)
ECCC	Emergency Care Coordination Center (ASPR)
EEC	Enterprise Executive Committee (PHEMCE)
EID	Emerging Infectious Diseases
EMT	Emergency Medical Technician
ESC	Enterprise Senior Council (PHEMCE)
EUA	Emergency Use Authorization
FDA	Food and Drug Administration
FFN	Fill-Finish Network
FY	Fiscal Year
GHSI	Global Health Security Initiative
GLP	Good Laboratory Practices
hBAT	heptavalent Botulinum Antitoxin
HHS	Department of Health and Human Services
HPP	Hospital Preparedness Program
IND	Investigational New Drug
IPT	Integrated Program Team (PHEMCE)
IRAT	Influenza Risk Assessment Tool
IV	Intravenous
LRN	Laboratory Research Network
MCM	Medical Countermeasure
MDR	Multi-Drug Resistant
MCMi	Medical Countermeasures Initiative (FDA)
MCMSI	Medical Countermeasures Strategic Investor
MIO	MCMSI Interface Office
MTA	Material Threat Assessment
MTD	Material Threat Determination
MVA	Modified Vaccinia Ankara
NBSB	National Biodefense Science Board
NDA	New Drug Application
NDMS	National Disaster Medical System
NGO	Non-Governmental Organization

NHSS	2009 National Health Security Strategy
NIAID	National Institute for Allergy and Infectious Diseases
NIOSH	National Institute for Occupational Safety and Health
NIH	National Institutes of Health
NIST	National Institute of Standards and Technology
NLM	National Library of Medicine
NPM	National Postal Model
OGA	Office of Global Affairs (HHS)
PAHPA	Pandemic and All-Hazards Preparedness Act
PAHPRA	Pandemic and All-Hazards Preparedness Reauthorization Act
PEP	Post-Exposure Prophylaxis
PHEMCE	HHS Public Health Emergency Medical Countermeasures Enterprise
PHPR	(CDC Office of) Public Health Preparedness and Response
POC	Point of Care
PPE	Personal Protective Equipment
REC	Regional Emergency Coordinator (ASPR)
rPA	Recombinant (anthrax) Protective Antigen
RPD	Respiratory Protective Device
RPE	Respiratory Protective Equipment
RPI	Relative Priority Index
SLEP	Shelf-Life Extension Program
SLTT	State, Local, Tribal, and Territorial
SNS	Strategic National Stockpile
SRF	Special Reserve Fund (Project BioShield)
TIC	Toxic Industrial Chemical
TRA	Terrorism Risk Assessment
TRLs	Technology Readiness Levels
USDA	U.S. Department of Agriculture
USG	United States Government
VA	U.S. Department of Veterans Affairs
VAERS	Vaccine Adverse Event Reporting System
VIG	Vaccinia Immune Globulin
VFC	Vaccines for Children (Infrastructure) (CDC)
VTEUs	Vaccine and Treatment Evaluation Units (NIH)
WHO	World Health Organization

APPENDIX 2. KEY NEAR-AND MID-TERM IMPLEMENTATION PLAN MILESTONES

This table summarizes select key milestones, identified in this plan, that are projected for completion within the next five years. This subset of milestones is not intended to be comprehensive. The Assistant Secretary for Preparedness and Response (ASPR) will establish an internal tracking mechanism to monitor and evaluate the execution of all priorities identified in the 2012 PHEMCE Implementation Plan and report progress regularly to senior PHEMCE leadership.

Table 4. Key Near- and Mid-Term Implementation Plan Milestones

Activity Number	Milestone Description	Lead Agency	Projected Completion Date
GOAL 1. Identify, create, develop, manufacture, and procure critical medical countermeasures.			
1.1.1	Lead PHEMCE partner agencies to define strategic end-states for all PHEMCE capabilities based on a clear description of the preparedness goals across the PHEMCE	ASPR	FY13
1.1.4	Implement PHEMCE-wide portfolio tracking tools to further enable coordinated planning and management of CBRN MCM development	ASPR	FY13
1.1.5	Consider expansion of the portfolio tracking tools to include pan flu or other EID portfolios as needed	ASPR	FY18
1.1.7	Further develop, implement, and evaluate the PHEMCE prioritization framework through the improvement of a suite of analytic decision support and visualization tools and models	ASPR	FY17
1.1.9	Further develop, implement, and evaluate the PHEMCE prioritization framework by assessing strengths and limitations of the framework components	ASPR	FY17
1.2.1	Formalize roles, responsibilities, policies,	DHS /	FY13

Activity Number	Milestone Description	Lead Agency	Projected Completion Date
	and procedures for conducting the next generation of MTAs and TRAs	HHS	
1.2.2	Develop updated disease assessments based on refinements to available data sources and modeling methodologies	BARDA	FY14
1.2.4	Develop or update MCM requirements for CBRN threats, as well as requirements that address multiple threats, as detailed in Objective 1.2	ASPR	FY14
1.2.5	Develop or update MCM requirements for CBRN threats, as detailed in Objective 1.2	ASPR	FY17
1.2.6	Develop capabilities-based requirements that capture MCM needs in broad areas, with a strong emphasis on end-user needs for biological diagnostics, CBRN therapeutics, prophylaxis for biological threats, and non-pharmaceutical MCM needs such as ventilators and respirators	ASPR	FY14
1.3.5	Develop candidates for a next generation anthrax vaccine, broad spectrum antiviral, influenza antiviral, and a next generation influenza vaccine to the stage where they can be considered for advanced development support.	NIH	FY17
1.3.7b	Acquire or maintain critical medical countermeasures as detailed in Table 3	BARDA / CDC	FY13
1.3.7c	Acquire or maintain critical medical countermeasures such as detailed in Table 3	BARDA / CDC	FY17
1.4.4	Establish a Clinical Research Organization (CRO) Network	BARDA	FY15
GOAL 2. Establish and communicate clear regulatory pathways to facilitate medical countermeasure development and use.			
2.1.2a1	Develop guidance for industry on developing multiplexed diagnostic devices	FDA	FY14
2.1.2b2	Develop guidance on establishing the performance of radiation biodosimetry	FDA	FY14
	devices		

Table 4. (Continued)

Activity Number	Milestone Description	Lead Agency	Projected Completion Date
2.1.5	Develop a partners program to link FDA scientists with extramural partners to pursue cutting edge regulatory science projects	FDA	FY14
GOAL 3. Develop logistics and operational plans for optimized use of medical countermeasures at all levels of response.			
3.1.2	Develop a risk-based analysis of investment needs by leveraging perspectives from the intelligence community and DHS risk assessment processes	CDC / DHS	FY14
3.1.7	Charge the National Biodefense Science Board (NBSB) and the Board of Scientific Counselors (BSC) to: Identify the anticipated responsibilities of the SNS in the year 2020 Recommend approaches for meeting those responsibilities as efficiently as possible Propose metrics for reporting program capability and informing improvement.	ASPR / CDC	FY13
3.2.4	Establish a process to validate laboratory methods and enhance national capacity to rapidly test clinical specimens and determine who has been exposed to biological agents	CDC	FY17
3.2.5	Develop rapid antimicrobial resistance testing to quickly identify agents that may be resistant to first-line MCMs in the SNS	CDC / DHS / DOD	FY17
3.2.6a	Develop national smallpox vaccine and anthrax response strategies	ASPR / CDC	FY13
3.2.6c	Develop an assessment of state and local capacity to utilize cytokines for ARS-associated neutropenia following use of an improvised nuclear device	ASPR / CDC	FY13
3.2.6d	Develop a decision-making and planning guidance for dispensing models to meet the diverse needs of communities	ASPR / CDC	FY14

Activity Number	Milestone Description	Lead Agency	Projected Completion Date
3.2.6e	Develop end-user handbook(s) for various stakeholders that will include: response strategies, MCM CONOPS, utilization guidance, and clinical practice information.	ASPR / CDC	Mid- to long-term
3.2.6f	Develop planning guidance for patient decontamination in a mass exposure chemical incident	ASPR / CDC	FY13
3.2.12	Develop and implement a strategic policy framework to respond to international requests for HHS public health emergency MCMs, and to accept assistance from foreign countries	ASPR	FY14
3.2.14	Work with Canada and Mexico to address barriers to providing mutual assistance and harmonizing utilization policies for MCMs during international public health emergencies under the framework of the U.S.-Canada Beyond the Border Initiative, and as called for in the North American Plan for Animal and Pandemic Influenza.	ASPR	FY15
3.3.1	Develop a comprehensive MCM messaging program and multi-year implementation plan	ASPR / CDC	FY15
3.4.1	Develop a comprehensive Action Plan for monitoring the safety and clinical benefit of MCMs during public health emergencies.	FDA / CDC	FY14
GOAL 4. Address medical countermeasure gaps for all sectors of the American civilian population.			
4.3.1	Provide clinicians with dosing and use guidance for applying stockpiled MCMs to pediatric populations, with the caveat that this guidance could only be used in an emergency (e.g., under an EUA)	ASPR / CDC	FY17
4.3.2	Ensure that public health and medical information distributed during public health emergencies is delivered in a manner that	ASPR / CDC	FY14

Table 4. (Continued)

Activity Number	Milestone Description	Lead Agency	Projected Completion Date
	takes into account the range of communication and other functional needs of the intended recipients, including at-risk individuals		
4.3.8	Integrate operational requirements, considerations, resources and action items for pediatric and other at-risk populations into ASPR Playbooks	ASPR	FY14
THREAT-BASED APPROACHES			
ANTHRAX			
T.A.1	Complete several stakeholder engagements and subject matter expert meetings to update anthrax clinical guidelines for all populations	CDC	FY14
T.A.2	Publish of an updated anthrax clinical guidance	CDC	FY14
T.A.3	Develop risk communication materials for an anthrax incident	CDC	FY14
T.A.6	Work with the anthrax vaccine manufacturer to support research into dose-sparing strategies for PEP vaccine use	NIH / CDC / FDA	FY13
T.A.9	Complete anthrax vaccine prioritization guidance	CDC	FY14
T.A.16	Support expansion of domestic manufacturing capacity for the currently licensed anthrax vaccine, to include: validating new manufacturing processes; conducting additional non-clinical and clinical studies; and pursuing licensure of a new facility	BARDA	FY17
OTHER BACTERIAL THREATS			
T.OB.2	Qualify animal efficacy models for anthrax, plague, and tularemia in support of PEP and treatment indications, through	NIH	FY14

Activity Number	Milestone Description	Lead Agency	Projected Completion Date
	the FDA's animal model qualification process		
T.OB.6	Develop animal models for testing MCMs against Burkholderia pseudomallei and Burkholderia mallei	BARDA	FY14
SMALLPOX			
T.S.1	Maintain sufficient quantities of smallpox vaccines in the SNS to provide a vaccination response capability for every American during a smallpox emergency, if appropriate	CDC / BARDA	FY14
T.S.4	Deliver to the SNS a subset of the required treatment courses of the smallpox antivirals currently under contract, with full delivery being completed in the mid term	BARDA	FY14 / FY17
PANDEMIC INFLUENZA			
T.PI.2	Ensure that all operational plans for pandemic influenza communication are updated, exercised, evaluated, and improved to facilitate effective communication strategies; develop an approach, definitions, tools and models for a risk communication response plan	CDC	FY17
T.PI.3	Maintain and update the existing stockpile of novel influenza virus and pre-pandemic vaccines and adjuvants, as needed	BARDA	FY14
T.PI.4	Develop rapid methods to produce candidate vaccine viruses that allow accelerated production of vaccine lots for eventual fill and finish by manufacturers. Complete work on development of rapid laboratory methods to expedite testing to determine the antigen content of influenza vaccine bulks and enable vaccine formulation prior to product fill and finish.	CDC / BARDA / FDA	FY14
T.PI.9	Support the development of novel recombinant vaccine candidates for both	BARDA	FY14

Table 4. (Continued)

Activity Number	Milestone Description	Lead Agency	Projected Completion Date
	pandemic and seasonal influenza through Phase II clinical trials		
T.PI.13	Award contracts for the advanced development of new influenza antiviral drugs	BARDA	FY14
T.PI.14	Expand surveillance for antiviral susceptibility	CDC	FY14
T.PI.15	Review and evaluate potential benefits and disadvantages of different antiviral use strategies, and reassess the quantity and composition of antiviral stockpiles by various levels of government and other partners, taking fiscal constraints and manufacturing capacity into account	CDC / NIH / BARDA / FDA	FY14
T.PI.16	Develop new plans for antiviral distribution and dispensing	CDC	FY14
T.PI.21	Commence development of new sequencing- based diagnostic assays and prototype device development for detection of influenza viruses and other respiratory pathogens	CDC / BARDA	FY14
T.PI.25	Work with federal and SLTT partners to implement guidance developed by the USG for situations in which limited vaccine availability requires targeted vaccination of persons with high-risk conditions	CDC	FY17
T.PI.27	Move several universal influenza vaccine candidates into early-phase human clinical testing	NIH	FY17
T.PI.28	Support at least one novel viral antigen or universal vaccine candidate expected to be evaluated in Phase II clinical studies in the mid term	BARDA	FY17
T.PI.30	Support advanced development of at least two drugs with novel mechanism(s) of action through Phase III clinical studies	BARDA	FY17

Activity Number	Milestone Description	Lead Agency	Projected Completion Date
RADIOLOGICAL AND NUCLEAR THREATS			
T.RN.7	Qualify rodent and non-human primate animal models for pivotal animal efficacy studies	NIH	FY17
T.RN.8	Finalize clinical guidance for MCMs to address radiation-induced neutropenia	CDC / ASPR	FY17
CAPABILITIES-BASED APPROACHES			
CBRN DIAGNOSTICS			
C.D.1	Initiate funding for the development of biological agent diagnostic systems, chemical agent diagnostic systems, and systems to identify and characterize unknown threats, including development of assays and instrumentation to address PHEMCE requirements for high-throughput and POC usage	NIH	FY14
C.D.5	Develop reference profile panels of threat agents that will support generation of requisite datasets required for licensure of a next-generation diagnostic platform	NIH	FY17
C.D.7	Develop and validate additional radionuclide bioassay diagnostic tests to allow rapid detection and measurement of radionuclides in clinical specimens	CDC	FY17
NON-PHARMACEUTICAL MEDICAL COUNTERMEASURES			
C.NP.4	Reassess the quantity and composition of respirator stockpiles for pandemic influenza and other threats, taking fiscal constraints into account, to determine whether the stockpiling of respirators in the SNS should be continued	CDC	FY14
C.NP.6	Develop an all-hazards ventilator assessment that will define both the quantities of ventilators for stockpiling and the desired device attributes for effectively responding to a range of lung injuries associated with different threat agents	ASPR	FY14

Table 4. (Continued)

Activity Number	Milestone Description	Lead Agency	Projected Completion Date
C.NP.7	Publish national planning guidance for conducting mass patient decontamination in a chemical incident	ASPR / DHS	FY14
C.NP.9	Initiate a research program to address critical knowledge gaps in the subject of patient decontamination	BARDA	FY14
CENTERS FOR INNOVATION IN ADVANCED DEVELOPMENT AND MANUFACTURING			
C.CIADM.2	Establish the CIADM governance structure	BARDA	FY14
C.CIADM.3	Construct and qualify CIADM infrastructure	BARDA	FY17
CROSS-CUTTING CAPABILITIES			
C.CC.1	Establish a Fill-Finish Network	BARDA	FY14
C.CC.3	Establish the MCMSI and MCMSI MIO	BARDA	FY14
C.CC.4	Establish a Visualization Hub to provide analytic decision support and access to real-time modeling capabilities to senior decision makers within ASPR and the PHEMCE	BARDA	FY14
C.CC.13	Establish an MCM advanced development and manufacturing facility	DoD	FY14
C.CC.14	Establish a dedicated biological safety level 4 laboratory capable of conducting GLP testing and evaluation of MCMs	DoD	FY17

End Notes

[1] Available at: http://www.phe.gov/Preparedness/mcm/phemce/Pages/strategy.aspx

[2] The PHEMCE mission components – requirement-setting; early-stage research; advanced development/manufacturing; regulatory science management; procurement/inventory management/stockpiling; response planning, policy, guidance, and communication; deployment/distribution/dispensing/administration; and monitoring/evaluation/assessment – are discussed in detail in the 2012 PHEMCE Strategy.

[3] Available at: http://www.phe.gov/Preparedness/mcm/phemce/Pages/strategy.aspx

4 Available at: http://www.phe.gov/Preparedness/planning/authority/nhss/strategy/Pages/ default.aspx

5 Available at http://www.phe.gov/Preparedness/planning/authority/nhss/ip/Pages/default.aspx

6 The high-priority threats identified in the 2012 PHEMCE Strategy, including all those determined by DHS to pose a material threat to national security, are anthrax, botulism, cyanide, emerging infectious diseases (including pandemic influenza), gram negative organisms (tularemia, plague, glanders, meliodosis, typhus), multi-drug resistant (MDR) anthrax, nerve agents, radiological agents, nuclear agents, smallpox, and viral hemorrhagic fevers (Marburg, Ebola).

7 End-users may include first responders, emergency room physicians and nurses and other facility-based caregivers, state and local emergency planners, public health officials, and others.

8 A product with an oral, nasal, or dermal delivery is easier to administer, in most circumstances, than an intravenous or intramuscular injection. In addition, in mass distribution schemes, there is a general benefit to limiting the number of times that provider-patient interaction is needed.

9 A product that is routinely used in medical practice will be more familiar to end-users in terms of both administration and appropriate use than one intended solely for use in emergencies.

10 In an ideal situation, all products procured for use during public health emergencies will be approved, licensed, or cleared by the FDA for their targeted population(s) and indication(s), in the formulation appropriate for their intended use. Approval, licensure, or clearance of a product enables the greatest flexibility and most timely access to MCMs in a public health emergency. However, in the absence of such an ideal situation, all efforts will be made to obtain sufficient safety and efficacy data to support use under the variety of other regulatory mechanisms that can allow for use of these products in an emergency, such as under an Emergency Use Authorization (EUA), or as part of a clinical trial or an expanded access program.

11 At-risk individuals have needs in one or more of the following functional areas: communication, medical care, maintaining independence, supervision, and transportation. At-risk groups may include children, senior citizens, and pregnant women, as well as people who have disabilities, live in institutionalized settings, are from diverse cultures, have limited English proficiency or are non-English speaking, are transportation-disadvantaged, have chronic medical disorders, or have pharmacological dependency. See http://www.phe.gov/preparedness/planning/abc/pages/default.aspx

12 The Public Health Emergency Medical Countermeasures Enterprise Review: Transforming the Enterprise to Meet Long-Range National Needs. August 2010. http://www.phe.gov/preparedness/mcm/enterprisereview/Pages/default.aspx

13 The PHEMCE reports annually on the status and formulary needs for all medical products stockpiled in the SNS, as required by the Pandemic and All-Hazards Preparedness Act and Homeland Security Presidential Directive-21.

14 TRAs are comprehensive, quantitative assessments of terrorism risk within a specified threat type (i.e., C-B-R-N) used to: inform investments; aid in identifying threats, vulnerabilities, and knowledge gaps; and support strategic risk management planning. DHS conducts four formal terrorism risk assessments: the Biological Terrorism Risk Assessment (BTRA), Chemical Terrorism Risk Assessment (CTRA), Integrated Terrorism Risk Assessment (ITRA), and Radiological/Nuclear Terrorism Risk Assessment (RNTRA).

15 MTAs are DHS-led assessments that project the number of individuals likely to be exposed to a threat agent in a plausible, high-consequence scenario.

[16] MTDs are issued by the Secretary of Homeland Security for threat agents deemed to pose a material threat sufficient to affect national security. The MTD is necessary, but not sufficient, to support a medical countermeasure acquisition under Project BioShield using the Special Reserve Fund (see Project BioShield, P.L. 108-276; available at: http://www.hsdl.org/?view&did=449237).

[17] Throughout the body of this Implementation Plan, activities that are led by the BARDA component of ASPR are so identified, while activities that involve BARDA in coordination with other ASPR components, or a predominant lead by these other components, are designated with an "ASPR" lead.

[18] Examples include FluAid and FluSurge. FluAid provides a range of estimates of impact in terms of deaths, hospitalizations, and outpatient visits due to pandemic influenza, while FluSurge predicts the surge in demand for hospital-based services during an influenza pandemic, yielding estimates of the number of hospitalizations (including ICU admissions) and deaths caused by a pandemic in comparison to existing hospital capacity.

[19] This includes all Category A, B, and C agents, including influenza.

[20] Under certain circumstances – when it is neither ethical nor feasible to conduct human efficacy studies – FDA may grant marketing approval based on adequate and well-controlled animal studies when the results of those studies establish that the drug or biological product is reasonably likely to produce clinical benefit in humans. Demonstration of the product's safety in humans is still necessary (21 CFR 314.600 for drugs; 21 CFR 601.90 for biological products).

[21] These include the nerve agents (sarin, VX, soman), and sulfur mustard.

[22] Such as cyanide, chlorine, and phosgene

[23] Such as parathion, chlorpyrifos, disulfoton, and the rodenticides sodium fluoroacetate, strychnine, and tetramethylenedisulfotetramine (TETS)

[24] Garcia, M, et al. Productive replication of Ebola virus is regulated by the c-Abl1 tyrosine kinase. 29 Feb 2012. Sci Transl Med. 4(123).

[25] For more information, see https://www.medicalcountermeasures.gov/federal-initiatives/guidance/about-the-trls.aspx

[26] These are therapies that reduce morbidity or mortality by targeting key host-cell molecules involved in immune-modulation, inflammation, and regulation of innate immunity.

[27] P.L. 108-276; available at: http://www.hsdl.org/?view&did=449237.

[28] These priorities include new products coming through the advanced development pipeline, as well as enhancements to current products in the SNS.

[29] Includes inventory held in both the SNS and alternative stockpiles

[30] Contingent upon available resources

[31] Assuming appropriations are available to maintain currently stockpiled and programmed levels

[32] Solicitations are ongoing to maintain existing preparedness levels and manufacturing capacity established under previous contracts.

[33] To Be Determined - Purchase of medical countermeasures under Project BioShield are planned pending appropriations

[34] DSNS refers to the Division of Strategic National Stockpile, the CDC division responsible for managing the SNS, whose mission is to deliver critical medical assets to the site of a national emergency.

[35] This includes antimicrobials for the following threat agents: anthrax, plague, tularemia, typhus, and secondary infections resulting from radiological and nuclear agents or pandemic influenza.

[36] Advanced development of this MCM class is not expected until the long-term, but early stage research is ongoing.

[37] The PHEMCE will also work with other federal partners with resources in this area, including the Advanced Manufacturing Partnership National Program Office recently established by the National Institute of Standards and Technology (NIST). More information is available at http://www.manufacturing.gov/welcome.html.

[38] For more information, see http://www.niaid.nih.gov/labsandresources/resources/Pages/default.aspx.

[39] More information on these Centers for Innovation in Advanced Development and Manufacturing can be found in the Capabilities- based Approaches section.

[40] FDA launched the MCMi in August 2010 in response to the 2010 PHEMCE Review and to build on the substantive MCM work ongoing at FDA. The MCMi mission is to promote the development of MCMs by enhancing FDA's regulatory processes and fostering the establishment of clear regulatory pathways for MCMs, and to facilitate timely access to available MCMs by establishing effective regulatory policies and mechanisms. For more information, see http://www.fda.gov/EmergencyPreparedness/MedicalCountermeasures/default.htm.

[41] FDA accomplishments under the MCMi are detailed in the MCMi annual status reports available at http://www.fda.gov/EmergencyPreparedness/MedicalCountermeasures/ ucm 270744.htm.

[42] More information on FDA's Action Teams can be found at http://www.fda.gov/Emergency Preparedness/MedicalCountermeasures/ucm263066.htm.

[43] FDA has developed a pre-EUA submission process whereby FDA works with product sponsors or government agencies, such as CDC, to develop pre-EUA packages prior to the declared emergency that may form the basis of an EUA request and issuance during a declared emergency. Pre-EUA packages contain data and other information about the safety and efficacy of an MCM, its intended use under an EUA, and information about the potential emergency situation that might unfold. The pre-EUA process allows FDA scientific and technical subject matter experts to begin a review of information and assist in the development of conditions for the authorization, fact sheets, and other documentation needed for an EUA in advance of an emergency. This advance work ensures the document is well- prepared for a potential EUA and significantly reduces the time needed during an emergency to review the submission and issue an EUA when appropriate. CDC develops pre-EUA packages (and IND applications) for submission to FDA for MCMs held in the SNS.

[44] More information on FDA's MCM Regulatory Science Program is available at http://www.fda.gov/EmergencyPreparedness/MedicalCountermeasures/ucm263071.htm.

[45] Topic areas for FDA's MCM Regulatory Science Program to date have included animal model development and qualification; identification and qualification of biomarkers for safety and efficacy; immune responses, including identification of correlates of protection; methods to assess product quality and related product release assays; risk communication to improve public health outcomes; validation of next-generation in vitro diagnostic platforms; assessment of the performance of emergency medical equipment; and real-time tracking and evaluation of MCM safety and performance during public health emergencies.

[46] A qualified DDT can be included in an IND or a New Drug Application (NDA)/Biologics License Application (BLA) submission without the need for FDA to reconsider and reconfirm the suitability of the DDT as long as there are (1) no serious study flaws; (2) no attempts to apply the DDT outside the qualified context of use; and (3) no new and

conflicting scientific facts not known at the time the qualification was determined. For more information, see http://www.fda.gov/Drugs/DevelopmentApprovalProcess/Drug DevelopmentToolsQualificationProgram/default.htm

[47] http://www.fda.gov/EmergencyPreparedness/MedicalCountermeasures/ucm263073.htm

[48] 42 U.S.C. 247d-6b(a)

[49] Homeland Security Presidential Directive-21

[50] Examples include the CHEMPACK program of more than 1,900 forward-placed caches of nerve agent antidotes held in local custody throughout the nation, and the SNS 12-Hour Push Packages, which are poised to support arrival anywhere in the nation within 12 hours of the federal decision to deploy SNS assets.

[51] The DoD/FDA Shelf Life Extension Program (SLEP) is a fee-for-service program used to defer drug replacement costs for large stockpiles of date-sensitive pharmaceuticals held in environmentally controlled locations by extending their shelf life beyond the manufacturer's original expiration date. The program is limited to DoD and selected federal agencies.

[52] The NBSB was established to provide expert advice and guidance to the HHS Secretary on scientific, technical, and other matters of special interest to HHS regarding activities to prevent, prepare for, and respond to adverse health effects of public health emergencies resulting from chemical, biological, nuclear, and radiological events, whether naturally occurring, accidental, or deliberate. See http://www.phe.gov/preparedness/legal/boards /nbsb/pages/default.aspx

[53] The BSC of the CDC Office of Public Health Preparedness and Response (PHPR) is chartered to advise the HHS Secretary, the CDC Director, and the PHPR Director concerning strategies and goals for preparedness programs and research; conduct peer-review of scientific programs; perform secondary reviews of research grants; and monitor PHPR's overall strategic direction and focus.

[54] Including clinical experts and state and local health officials

[55] As may occur following, for example, use of an improvised nuclear device.

[56] The NPM program will continue to focus on the distribution of doxycycline (antibiotic) to U.S. Postal Service (USPS) employees in selected regions to enhance preparedness against anthrax. The intent of providing these employees pre-distributed packages of antibiotics is to increase their ability and willingness to participate in larger efforts to distribute MCMs to an affected community following an anthrax attack.

[57] See http://www.phe.gov/preparedness/planning/hpp/Pages/default.aspx

[58] See http://www.ghsi.ca/english/index.asp

[59] See http://www.dhs.gov/beyond-border-shared-vision-perimeter-security-and-economic-competitiveness

[60] See http://www.phe.gov/Preparedness/international/Documents/napapi.pdf

[61] Available at: http://www.phe.gov/nhss.

[62] For example, recent NBSB recommendations to pursue gathering of pre-event safety data on MCM use in children has been referred to the Presidential Commission for the Study of Bioethical Issues for further debate and resolution at the time of this writing.

[63] Pediatric populations refer to individuals under the age of 21 years.

[64] Public summary available at: http://www.phe.gov/Preparedness/planning/abc/Documents/ 2011-children-disasters.pdf

[65] See http://cybercemetery.unt.edu/archive/nccd/20110427002908/http:/www.children and dis asters.acf.hhs.gov/index.html

[66] The Animal Health Protection Act of 2002 defines the term "animal" as any member of the animal kingdom (except a human).

[67] See http://www.onehealthinitiative.com/

[68] Regional Emergency Coordinators (RECs) serve as ASPR's primary representatives throughout the country at the regional level. For more information, see http://www.phe.gov /Preparedness/responders/rec/Pages/default.aspx

[69] Information regarding respiratory protective devices for influenza needs is addressed in the capabilities-based approaches section.

[70] The target for noninstitutionalized adults aged 18 to 64 years is 80% with completion projected in 2020. For more information, see http://www.healthypeople.gov/2020/topics objectives 2020/objectiveslist.aspx?topicId=23

[71] More information on patient decontamination efforts is described in the Capabilities-Based Approaches section below as a non-pharmaceutical MCM. NIH will focus research efforts on highly toxic chemicals of greatest public health concern.

[72] See http://www.cdc.gov/niosh/npptl/topics/respirators/disp part/RespSource.html

[73] This assessment includes analysis of the ancillary supplies and infrastructure needs (e.g., power sources, oxygen gas demand) to operate mechanical ventilators.

[74] For more information, see https://www.medicalcountermeasures.gov/ barda/manu facturing. aspx

INDEX

A

B

C

D

O

P

R

S

T

U

V

W

Y